The Ultimate pH Solution

*Balance Your Body Chemistry
to Prevent Disease and Lose Weight*

Michelle Schoffro Cook
DNM, DAC, CNC

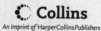
Collins
An Imprint of HarperCollinsPublishers

To my husband, Curtis.

THE ULTIMATE pH SOLUTION.
Copyright © 2008 by Michelle Schoffro Cook. All rights reserved. Printed in the United States of America. No part of this book may be used or reproduced in any manner whatsoever without written permission except in the case of brief quotations embodied in critical articles and reviews. For information, address HarperCollins Publishers, 10 East 53rd Street, New York, NY 10022.

HarperCoilins books may be purchased for educational, business, or sales promotional use. For information, please write: Special Markets Department, HarperCollins Publishers, 10 East 53rd Street, New York, NY 10022.

FIRST EDITION

Designed by Susan MacGregor

Library of Congress Cataloging-in-Publication Data has been applied for.

ISBN 978-0-06-133643-0

10 11 12 ❖/RRD 10 9 8 7 6

Contents

Foreword

For close to four decades, I have been studying the role that nutrition plays in life-long health and disease prevention. This research began as a personal journey to overcome a devastating stomach disorder that plagued my early life. Not only did the information I learned free me from my painful condition, it also wound up saving my life from the deadly effects of being exposed to Agent Orange while serving in Vietnam. I learned that food and nutrition choices are powerful allies in the fight against disease and poor health.

My healing journey became public with the publication of *Fit For Life* in 1985. I realized that I needed to share with the world the powerful knowledge I had gained from years of nutritional research. Food is, and always will be, our best medicine. Yet, in our modern world of processed, packaged, and artificially altered dining choices, food has become one of our worst enemies. The diseases of affluence—heart disease, cancer, osteoporosis, and obesity—have reached epidemic proportions. Instead of providing fuel for the complex and critical functions that keep our bodies and minds healthy, the modern, overly acidic diet that dominates our eating lifestyle is wreaking havoc on the delicate balance Michelle Schoffro Cook describes in *The Ultimate pH Solution*.

Michelle and I share many similarities on our healing journeys. She too began to study nutrition as medicine to overcome serious health problems. She has close to two decades of research and experience with her own health and that of her clients and patients. Over the years I have known Michelle, she has exhibited a resolute dedication and commitment to health and well-being, not only for herself but also for others who are deserving of life-saving information. What began as a private quest for health has become a mission to share with her readers the unparalleled importance of maintaining the crucial acid–alkaline balance within the body. Michelle does not simply tell you why it is important to balance your pH; she provides you with an intelligent game plan for success that includes simple, delicious recipes and easy lifestyle changes to help you in your quest for well-being. She is an active partner on your journey as you improve your health.

In my nearly forty years of research, I can identify a handful of essential concepts that are universal—that apply to everyone seeking health, energy, and a long life. Maintaining a proper pH balance is one of these essential concepts. Michelle has succeeded in simplifying this biochemical mystery while capturing its paramount significance to overall health and well-being. She has created an engaging, entertaining, and easy-to-use tool for anyone wishing to experience vibrant health and energy. Whether you are overcoming disease and disability or simply wishing to carry your good health long into the future, *The Ultimate pH Solution* will show you the way. It is a landmark book that all who are interested in their health, and the health of their loved ones, should read. While debunking long-held myths about pH balancing, Michelle Schoffro Cook clearly delineates the simple ways you can acquire and maintain the proper acid–alkaline balance in your blood. Follow *The Ultimate pH Solution* and you will be well on your way to a life free of pain, ill health, and disease—to a life dominated by health and well-being.

HARVEY DIAMOND
author of *Fit For Life*

Introduction

"The first wealth is health."

—RALPH WALDO EMERSON

I am about to tell you the secret to lasting health. It's so little known that even many doctors, nutritionists, and other health experts are unaware of it, though it is the one thing that is guaranteed to improve your health.

It's not about popping pills or eating more protein.

It's not about counting calories, carbs, or fat grams.

It's not about genetic predispositions to certain illnesses or conditions.

Once you know this one vital secret, you will hold the power to create—and maintain—your own good health. Imagine equipping your body with the tools it needs to ward off cold and flu viruses, heart disease, arthritis, osteoporosis, diabetes, kidney disease, and cancer. And as a bonus, you'll have more energy and feel better than ever, and excess weight will simply "melt off."

These days, many health "experts" are so busy telling people to get enough protein, vitamins, minerals, exercise, and so on to lose weight and feel healthy that they miss a factor that is far more critical to your health.

Adiós, Atkins!

Move over, Hamptons!

Step aside, South Beach!

Now you can stop following senseless diets that will only end up compromising your health.

Are you ready for the secret to permanently great health? Here it is: *Balance the pH level of your blood!*

What's pH, and why is it so important? Your pH level is the balance between acid and alkaline in your blood. An acidic pH level is not the same as acid reflux—when stomach acids needed for digestion flow back up the digestive tract, causing an acidic, burning sensation. Acid reflux is frequently

1

the result of poor food choices or combinations, or is brought on by reclining too soon after a meal. The acid I'm referring to is a subtle balance in your blood that can affect your whole body.

Imagine that acid and alkaline are two teams in a tug-of-war contest, each one holding the end of a long rope and trying to shift the balance to its side, and you'll have a good sense of what happens every single second in your body. When your pH balance tips toward either the acidic or the alkaline side of the spectrum, you are vulnerable to a variety of health problems. In North America, because of our current eating habits, it is rare for anyone to become excessively alkaline; excessive acid is much more common, as this book will explain.

Acidic blood is the precursor to almost every disease. Therefore, whether your blood is acidic or alkaline will determine whether you are susceptible to diseases such as cancer, arthritis, and heart disease. By "kicking acid" in your blood, you'll ward off diseases of all kinds, feel abundant energy, and shed excess pounds. Sound too good to be true? Believe it: these benefits have been proven by recognized medical journals.

There are no blood tests required to start benefiting from what I call the Kick Acid program. If you choose to check your pH (and I encourage you to do so), you'll find pH test paper at your local health food store. In chapter 2, I'll explain how to use it. If you're like most people, you'll be surprised to learn how acidic your body is. And while balancing pH may sound complicated, you're about to learn how simple it actually is.

As you read this book, you will learn the many health rewards of kicking acid. But to whet your appetite, here are just a few:

- Most of the diseases that plague people in the West could not occur in a pH-balanced body.
- The rate at which you age is determined by how acidic your blood is. Graying hair and wrinkling and sagging skin are all worsened by acid in your body.
- The reason cholesterol levels soar is to repair the damage caused to arteries by acidic blood, which scours your arterial walls like an S.O.S. pad.
- Cancer cells require acidity to survive. That's right: they thrive in an acid environment but are unable to survive in an alkaline one.
- Most people would experience significantly less pain if their pH was balanced. That includes those who suffer from serious disorders such as arthritis and fibromyalgia.

Put simply, if you want great health, alkalize your body. That means making it less acidic and more alkaline. Don't worry: you don't need to understand chemistry to reap the amazing health rewards of a more alkaline body.

I've spent almost two decades researching the latest health trends, seeking out information that helps restore health, and trying to find the secrets of lasting health. Along the way, I've observed that the incidence of chronic diseases such as cancer, heart disease, and arthritis is skyrocketing. I find it interesting that this is happening at a time in our historical evolution when there is tremendous access to so-called modern medicine.

It is also interesting that considerably more than half the population of both the United States and Canada is overweight or obese. This is largely due to the market growth of the fast-food and prepared-food industries, a growth mirrored by our expanding girth and our increased susceptibility to diseases. I'll explain more about the effects of fast food in the coming chapters.

I have long believed that Mother Nature, not the pharmaceutical giants, holds the key to great health. After nearly two decades of research, I am more convinced of that than ever. Indeed, offerings from Mother Nature can prevent disease, relieve pain, aid weight loss, provide abundant energy, and ensure vibrant health. This book will show you how to unlock her secrets to lasting health and vitality.

In *The Ultimate pH Solution*, you'll learn why making your blood more alkaline, and therefore alkalizing your whole body, makes all the difference between poor health and great health. You'll discover simple alkalizing techniques that take five minutes or less. These techniques will significantly alter your body's pH from acidic to slightly alkaline to help you restore balance and prevent disease.

While you're working toward alkalizing your body, you can still eat your favorite foods—steak, burgers, pasta, chocolate—on occasion. You'll simply be making a few small changes to your lifestyle and the way you eat. You'll find, as many others have found, that these changes are easy to make and, with minimal effort, fit into virtually any lifestyle.

After reading *The Ultimate pH Solution* you'll understand how

- Eating the right food alongside your favorite foods substantially minimizes the damage done by these acidic foods.
- Hopping into a luxurious bath can make your blood more alkaline (you just need to add the right ingredient, one that not only softens your skin but eliminates acid buildup in your tissues).
- Drinking more alkaline water can help ward off pain and inflammation linked to acidity.

- Eating more alkaline fruits and vegetables can help melt off excess weight.
- Adding a single ingredient to your water and drinking it throughout the day can give you more energy and help you overcome serious health problems.

Kicking acid and beating disease really can feel that good and be that simple. Yet, surprisingly, most people have never heard of this life-changing concept. What's more, many people are caught up in eating a high-protein diet or following some other fad diet, a sure-fire way to unbalance your pH and make you vulnerable to many diseases.

Let's consider osteoporosis, a disease that currently affects more than 25 million Americans and an estimated 1.4 million Canadians. There is plenty of research to show that the high protein content of meat and dairy products turns the blood acidic. Your bones act like bank accounts, storing the alkaline mineral calcium. Whenever your blood becomes acidic, your body makes calcium withdrawals from your bones to neutralize the acidity. If you're not depositing enough calcium from your diet into your bones, the calcium bank account in your bones will be overdrawn. This often results in osteoporosis.

Once you've balanced your pH, you'll find that most of your health problems will improve or disappear altogether. In chapter 3, you'll learn about the exciting medical and scientific research that supports the acid–disease connection. And throughout this book, you'll read about people just like you who kicked acid and successfully overcame their health issues. You'll discover, for example, how Gordon banished chronic seasonal allergies, Barbara beat fibromyalgia, Ray lost weight he'd struggled with for years, and Kirk boosted his immune system and stopped getting every cold and flu going around. All of these people are enjoying the tremendous results of balancing their body chemistry—and you can too!

It is my hope that, by reading *The Ultimate pH Solution*, you will gain a sense of empowerment and control over your health and life, and will understand how simple choices you make every day can help you live longer and live a better quality of life. It is also my hope that by implementing the suggestions in *The Ultimate pH Solution* you will live a life free from heart disease, osteoporosis, arthritis, diabetes, cancer, and other painful or life-threatening diseases.

Keep reading for the secret to lasting health, energy, immunity, and vitality!

CHAPTER 1

The Fatal Flaws in Our Standard American Diet (SAD)

"Tell me what you eat, I'll tell you who you are."

—JEAN ANTHELME BRILLAT-SAVARIN

For thousands of years, our human ancestors lived completely off the land. Their lives depended on their understanding of and connection to nature. Archeological evidence shows that they foraged for wild berries, seeds, nuts, and herbs; researchers estimate that approximately 95 percent of their diet consisted of these foods. To a much lesser extent, they also ate the meat of wild animals. Our hunter-gatherer ancestors subsisted in this way until the agricultural revolution, which started around 10,000 years ago. Over the following centuries, some hunter-gatherer and fishing societies moved to a life of farming and animal domestication. Even after 10,000 years of agriculture, some experts suggest that our bodies are still struggling to adapt to our change in diet from wild berries, greens, and animals to more domesticated animals and cultivated grains.

There is now a far more dangerous revolution taking place even as you read this book. It has the power to wreak havoc on us, damaging our bodies so they are vulnerable to countless diseases and obesity. This revolution was created by industrialization and the commercialization of our food supply.

Over the past 100 years or so, we have denatured our food supply more than ever before during human history and throughout our evolution. We've sprayed produce with chemicals originally derived from leftover toxic nerve agents when there was no longer a military use for them. We unleash mutant "ghost bugs"—bacteria shells filled with pesticides and injected with viruses— onto our food to kill insects that might dare take a few bites of *our* produce. Instead of depending on the natural mineralization of soil that occurs over time as Mother Nature composts decaying matter, we add artificially created chemical fertilizers. We even alter the genetic material of seeds before planting them, with the arrogant belief that we can improve upon what nature has created. We subject our food to radiation that destroys its life force in favor of an extended shelf life. To further prolong food's shelf life, its so-called attractiveness, and ultimately the business cycle during which companies can profit from selling it, we add synthetic chemicals in the form of colors; preservatives; stabilizers; flavors and flavor enhancers; ripening gases; waxes; conditioners; firming agents; heavy metals; nutrient "enrichers"; bleach; texturizers; and chemically altered fats, sugars, and amino acids that bear no resemblance to the food molecules they originated from. Mother Nature is marginalized from our food supply in favor of big business, food technologists, and corporate profit margins.

What we call "food" has few of the building blocks of life left in it. Based on our current understanding of nutrition, we know that food should contain several dozen vitamins and minerals, plentiful amounts of enzymes to aid in digestion, hundreds of phytochemicals (natural plant nutrients and pigments) that slow aging and prevent disease processes, fiber, amino acids, natural sugars, and essential fatty acids—all of which our bodies *require* to create healthy cells. Our bodies need healthful sugars from complex carbohydrates for the energy production required by every cell. We need amino acids from healthy and digestible proteins to build new tissues and organs. We require essential fatty acids from the fats found in vegetables, seeds, and nuts to protect our brains and nervous systems and ensure healthy immune systems that can fight off illness. We need enzymes to ensure healthy digestion of all these foods so our bodies will have the building blocks they require for healthy cell formation. These healthy cells create healthy tissues. Healthy tissues create healthy organs. Healthy organs create healthy organ systems. And healthy organ systems create healthy human bodies.

So it should come as no surprise that denatured food creates disease-prone, disease-laden, and overweight bodies. Even cooking food at temperatures higher than 118°F destroys its enzyme content. Yet millions continue to eat denatured food as part of the Standard American Diet (SAD).

The Standard American Diet truly is SAD when it comes to preventing disease and maintaining great health. Our excessive consumption of fast food, sugar, trans fats, meat, and food additives is the fast track to disease. We need to make simple changes to break free of the Standard American Diet or risk suffering one or more of the many diseases linked to it, including obesity, heart disease, brain disease, and many forms of cancer.

Don't worry: I'm not suggesting that you give up all of your favorite foods or pursue a vegetarian diet. You can still enjoy your favorites on occasion;

you just need to know simple tricks to restore the balance, tricks you'll learn later in this book.

But first, let's take a look at the components (and deficiencies) of the typical North American diet.

SWEET NOTHINGS

The average person consumes 150 pounds of refined sugar per year, which is astronomical in contrast to the 5 pounds per year our grandparents or great-grandparents ate at the turn of the 20th century. That's 30 times more sugar every year! While there are some inherent and well-known problems associated with refined sugar consumption (which you will learn more about in chapter 5), sugar is also extremely acid-forming in our bodies. Our sugar addiction has severe ramifications, none of which is particularly sweet.

Refined sugar is one of the worst poisons we put into our bodies. It can block our immune response for between four and six hours, lowering our natural defenses and making us less capable of fighting viruses, bacteria, and other pathogens. Sugar makes our bodies' pH very acidic, and with the average North American consuming 150 pounds of sugar annually, that's a great deal of acidity to overcome. It's not surprising that research has linked sugar to cancer, hormonal disruptions, arthritis, osteoporosis, cataracts, and many other degenerative diseases.

The manner in which sugar is processed exacerbates the problem. More than 60 chemicals are used in the processing of natural sugarcane's thick beige stalks into the fine, white granular product found in grocery stores and used in most baked goods and the vast majority of our foods. Many of these chemicals, including bleaches and deodorizers, are still present in the final product. At the same time, the naturally occurring minerals and vitamins found in the sugarcane plant are completely removed. The nutrients that are depleted are the more alkaline portion of sugarcane.

If this has you thinking about artificial sweeteners such as aspartame and saccharin, think again. These chemical cocktails are worse than refined sugar, and your body was not designed to break them down and properly remove them.

Sugar lurks in many unexpected places: it is used as an additive in foods ranging from meat to ketchup to salt. In chapter 4, I will help you eliminate the hidden sources of sugar from your diet. I'm not going to suggest that you cut all sweets from your diet. A small amount of sugar is not worrisome. But cutting out hidden sources of sugar and switching to more natural options can make a huge difference in balancing your body chemistry. In chapter 8, I'll teach you delicious and healthier options for satisfying your sweet tooth, including my favorite recipe for chocolate mousse!

FAUX FOOD

Sugar isn't the only food additive you need to be concerned about. Chemicals added to an endless list of both processed and "unprocessed" foods contribute to the acidity levels in our bodies. Food additives are supposed to "improve" the flavor, color, and commercial appeal of foods, thus increasing sales. They are also used to prolong shelf life. Unfortunately, there are a few serious problems with these chemicals:

1. Synthetic fillers are no replacement for nutrient-dense, fiber-rich, alkalizing foods such as vegetables, yet they are playing a larger and larger role in the typical North American diet.
2. In recent studies, many coloring agents, preservatives, synthetic flavors, and other chemicals have been found to be toxic to our bodies. Further research—unbiased research that's not funded by the food processing industry, that is—will likely prove that the vast majority, if not all, of these additives are toxic.
3. While research on the acid-forming effects of food additives is still in its infancy, I believe that many additives have a negative effect on the acid–base balance of your body once they are ingested.

When I talk to my patients about nutrition, I frequently ask them how many pounds of chemical food additives they eat in a year. I rarely get an answer above 5 pounds, because most people cannot fathom consuming 5 pounds of chemicals. They are shocked by the real numbers: research shows that the average person consumes 124 pounds of food chemicals per year. I'm not talking about vitamins and minerals or other nutrients, or even sugar. We eat 124 pounds a year of synthetic preservatives, colors, and many other artificial chemicals, none of which the human body was designed to handle. Nor did we have to deal with them for thousands of years of our evolution. As recently as a hundred years ago, there were no artificial chemicals; our ancestors' diet would not have included any of these predominantly acid-forming, toxic substances.

That disturbing amount is not really surprising when you consider how much of our food contains synthetic ingredients. In a typical packed lunch, you might find a roast beef sandwich with mayo and mustard on a white flour bun, an apple, potato chips, a couple of cookies, and maybe a thermos of coffee or a soda. What you don't see are the linalyl benzoate, monosodium glutamate, nitrates, sulfites, Yellow No. 5 or FD&C Blue No. 1. Sounds appetizing, doesn't it? To me, it sounds like the laboratory concoction Dr. Frankenstein might have thrown together to create his protégé-gone-wrong. Or maybe the mysterious concoction Dr. Jekyll drank to transform into his evil alter ego, Mr. Hyde.

There are more than 3,000 additives and preservatives in our food supply today.[1] Sugar, salt, pepper, and even foods such as mustard can be classified as additives; however, the vast majority of these hidden ingredients are chemicals that act as coloring agents, artificial flavors and flavor enhancers, stabilizers, conditioners, thickeners, bleaching agents, preservatives, and pesticides. These are hardly ingredients you would intentionally add to your grocery list.

Food additives are a controversial topic. Proponents say testing—usually by government departments such as the U.S. Food and Drug Administration (FDA) or Health Canada—is adequate to determine safety and that the amounts are so small they could not possibly harm humans. My reply is threefold. First, we are only now beginning to see the long-term health hazards of many supposedly safe additives. Neither industry-led nor independent short-term studies on animals or even trials on human subjects can accurately forecast these hazards. There are very few long-term studies of this nature. Second, there are virtually no studies examining the combined effects of two or more of these additives, yet we are exposed to them in combination on a regular basis. Third, a poison is still a poison, no matter how small the quantity. The body must still deal with it as a toxic substance and redirect energy toward a solution. That small quantity, day after day, month after month, year after year, is equivalent to water dripping on the hardest stone. Eventually, it will wear the stone down.

While not a food additive, a common toxin known as bisphenol A provides a useful comparison for our exposure to chemicals. In a recent article in Canada's *Globe and Mail* newspaper on the toxic effects of bisphenol A, journalist Martin Mittelstaedt stated: "At the heart of the intense debate over bisphenol A is that it challenges the main tenet of modern toxicology, the idea that the dose makes the poison, a principle credited to the 15th-century Swiss alchemist Theophrastus Paracelsus."[2] Since the 1980s, regulators have allowed the use of this chemical in aluminum cans, hard plastic beverage bottles, baby bottles, dental sealants, and many other consumer products. They insisted that the amount of bisphenol A finding its way into our food and ultimately into our bodies wasn't high enough to cause damage. But more recent testing demonstrates that bisphenol A mimics human hormones and that a minuscule amount of the toxin is sufficient to cause serious damage, even if substantially larger exposures have no effects. The petrochemical–derived substance has been linked with early onset of puberty, declining sperm counts, miscarriages, ovarian dysfunction, and massive increases in breast and prostate cancer.[3]

Keep in mind that bisphenol A is only one of thousands of chemicals to which we are exposed. And we are just beginning to see the effects in the form of skyrocketing rates of disease.

I could go on at length about the dangers of food additives in our diet. The ones mentioned in the box on pages 10 to 12 are just a sampling. With more than 3,000 different chemicals added to our food, the discussion of the health repercussions could be endless. And neither the FDA nor Health Canada has done sufficient testing on the majority of these additives. Not nearly enough is known about their effects on growing children, immune-compromised individuals, or the elderly. Almost no testing has been done to determine the health repercussions of a lifelong exposure to food additives, or of combining two or more chemicals.

An increasing number of studies have found that many of these chemicals have disastrous effects on our body, yet we've really just hit the tip of the iceberg. I believe that, over time, we'll see more and more research added to the volume of scientific data showing that food additives have dangerous health effects. While the research continues, suffice it to say that the fewer additives in your diet, the less potential risk you run.

COMMON FOOD ADDITIVES

Artificial colors: There is no nutritional value in artificial colors. Worse still, these ingredients often take the place of those that *do* have nutritional value. For example, their presence in fruit juice often signals that little to no fruit is contained in the juice. Artificial colors have been linked with cancers and hyperactivity disorders in children. (You may recall that the FDA recommended a ban on Red Dye No. 3 in the 1980s but the federal administration overruled the recommendation.)

Preservatives: Nitrates and sulfites are two common categories of preservatives. Nitrates are used in many meats (bacon, hot dogs, pastrami, and bologna, for example) as a curing agent, to preserve color, and to reduce bacteria. Nitrates are particularly damaging when they convert to nitrites—either through cooking or during digestion, when they combine with amines to form N–nitroso compounds.

These compounds are known carcinogens, linked to cancer of the mouth, brain, stomach, esophagus, and bladder.

Sulfites are chemicals used to keep produce looking fresh and to prevent discoloration. They occur naturally in some foods and in wine, although many wineries use additional sulfites to preserve their wines. (Organic wines usually have fewer—and only naturally occurring—sulfites.) In the mid-1980s, the FDA banned the use of sulfites on most fruits and vegetables and in salad bars, in response to growing evidence linking them to severe allergic reactions, including fatalities. However, they are still used on dried fruit and in packaged foods.

Sugar substitutes, or replacement sweeteners: These come with many names—from saccharin (which the FDA tried unsuccessfully to ban 30 years ago) to aspartame and sucralose—and many claims, but all are best avoided. If you don't recognize the chemical names, some of the brand names include Sweet'N Low, Sugar Twin, NutraSweet, Equal, Sunnett, Sweet One, and Splenda. Some of the negative symptoms caused by these artificial sweeteners include headaches, dizziness, and nausea, and a lengthy list of serious diseases has been linked to their use.

While the problems with refined sugar are many, the problems with sugar substitutes are potentially greater. Let's consider aspartame, otherwise known as NutraSweet or Equal. Aspartame is 90 percent amino acids (aspartic acid and phenylalanine) and 10 percent methanol, which is also known as wood alcohol or methyl alcohol. A single 12-ounce soft drink sweetened with aspartame can contain up to 30 milligrams of methanol. Methanol is toxic to the human body because we do not have the necessary enzymes to break it down (more on the importance of enzymes later). Instead, our bodies convert methanol into formaldehyde, a known carcinogen, and ultimately into formic acid, or formate, which creates excess acidity in our bodies. Scientific studies link aspartame consumption to many diseases and disorders, including anxiety, brain tumors, birth defects, depression, epilepsy, migraines, psychiatric disorders, premenstrual syndrome, and reproductive problems.[4]

Pesticides: It's difficult to reconcile pesticides with food ingredients, considering that pesticides are intended to kill. A common class of pesticides called organophosphates was derived from nerve agents developed for use during the First World War. When the war was over, industry adapted these toxins for a new commercial application: pesticides to spray on our food supply! While we may be aware that we are ingesting the residue of pesticides when we eat non-organic fruits and vegetables, they are also commonly used on the grains that find their way into our breads, cereals, and baked goods.

Ethyl formate: Used in the food industry as a flavor enhancer as well as a fungicide and larvicide for cereals and dried fruits, ethyl formate also goes by the name formic acid—sound familiar? In large quantities, it can cause not only excess acidity, but also blindness.[5]

Gelatin, or gelatine: Essentially an animal protein product, gelatin is used in food as a stabilizer, thickener, and texturizer. In the case of Jell-O, the gelatin is made of collagen from the bones, hooves, and connective tissues of pigs or cows. These ingredients are treated with strong acid or alkaline substances to break them down into gelatin, which is then combined with artificial colors and flavors to create a toxic treat. Acidic on its own, gelatin is often found in acidic foods such as ice cream, cheese, and margarine. Gelatin has no nutritional value and should be avoided.

Polysorbate 80: Commercially known as Tween 80, polysorbate 80 is used in the food industry as an emulsifier (basically, a thickening agent). It is created from sorbitol (an acidic sugar alcohol) and oleic acid (which is a healthy fatty acid when it is not chemically altered and combined with other ingredients).

Monosodium glutamate (MSG): One of the most common and devastating additives found in our food, MSG increases acidity in our bodies. Research on the toxic effects of MSG in its many disguises is substantial and warrants an entire book on its own. Adverse health effects range from headaches and migraines to asthma, breathing difficulties, and digestive troubles, to name a few. Do yourself a favor and avoid this additive at any cost.

SALT OF THE EARTH

The diet of our pre-agricultural ancestors was rich in salt—not the salt now found on almost every table in small glass shakers, but potassium alkali salts, which are found in abundance in non-grain plant foods. These salts were eaten in their naturally occurring form. The salt we know today (and which some people love, to their detriment) is processed sodium chloride (NaCl), an addictive and overly used substance found in virtually every food choice in the Standard American Diet. Our SAD diet is also dangerously low in potassium alkali salts. Sodium chloride is acid-forming; potassium salts are not. The combination of a sodium chloride excess with a potassium deficiency further contributes to the acid load on our systems.

FAT, FAT, AND MORE FAT

In addition to large quantities of chemicals, sugar, and sugar substitutes, the average person eats excessive amounts of harmful saturated and trans fats and few or no beneficial fats (monounsaturated and polyunsaturated fats). Saturated fat, found primarily in animal products such as meat, poultry, and dairy products, has an acidifying effect on our bodies and offers no nutritional value.

We also eat high amounts of rancid and overheated oils in processed, packaged, and prepared foods, fried foods, cooking oils, margarine, shortening, and lard. While healthy fats are found in fresh, raw fruit and vegetables, nuts, seeds, and grains, as well as in oils derived from these ingredients, oils in our diet are typically rancid because they are old, have been processed incorrectly, have been exposed to light or oxygen for too long, or have been heated. Unfortunately, during the manufacturing process of most oils, the grains and seeds from which the oils are derived are stored for excessive amounts of time and are exposed to both light and oxygen. Worse, most oils are heated to over 500°F during their processing—even before they get to the grocery store shelves. That amount of heat turns almost all oils rancid. Of course, frying has the same effect on the oil.

Every oil has a different smoke point—the temperature after which it is no longer healthy and begins to smoke. Some oils, such as flaxseed oil, have a very low smoke point and, as a result, should never be heated. Olive oil smokes at just under 325°F, while macadamia nut oil reaches its smoke point at around 410°F, allowing you to cook with it at higher temperatures without destroying the health benefits of the oil (unless the oil has been overheated during manufacturing). When oils become rancid or overheated, the beneficial fatty acids break down into other compounds such as hydrocarbons, ketones, and aldehydes, all of which can raise the acidity of our bodies.

The average person also eats 5 pounds of trans fats per year. While there are different ways to turn a healthy fat into a trans fat, the vast majority of trans fats in our diet are artificially created by the food processing industry. Processing plants add hydrogen atoms to healthy fats to "saturate" the oil molecule, turning an unsaturated oil molecule into a saturated one. While this hydrogenation process may extend the shelf life of the oil, it destroys its healthful properties. Trans fats have been linked with countless diseases, and some places, such as New York City, are starting to ban them. I refer to these disease agents as "plastic fats" because they have absolutely no place in the human body. Trans fats are a relatively new phenomenon and certainly would not have had a role in our ancestors' diets even 100 years ago. Yet we are eating plentiful amounts of them. Trans fats and other harmful fats inflict damage on your body and increase its already overwhelming acid burden.

A diet high in these harmful fats increases the strain on the liver, an important and overworked detoxification organ that already has more than 500 other functions. Our intestines cannot break down or absorb poor-quality fats, so they must neutralize them with alkaline bile, a substance secreted by the liver. The bile combines with fats to form masses that are eliminated in the stool. Unfortunately, as our bodies try to neutralize these fats, much-needed calcium, sodium, and potassium are eliminated as well. These alkaline minerals perform many tasks in the body, including balancing excessive acids (which you will learn more about in chapter 2). If they are depleted to deal with bad fats, other bodily functions may be compromised.

The typical diet, if it contains any beneficial essential fatty acids at all, usually includes omega-6 fatty acids from nuts, seeds, and grains. Omega-6 fatty acids are found in the highest concentrations in corn, sunflower, and safflower oils, and in the meat of animals fed these foods. These oils are present in many packaged foods and baked goods, and are frequently used as the basis of vegetable oils or margarine. Most people do not get adequate amounts of omega-3 fatty acids, which are found in flaxseeds, flaxseed oil, and fatty fish such as salmon, mackerel, and cod.

Both types of fatty acids are essential to a healthy body: they help to regulate blood pressure and blood clotting; they ensure that our immune and inflammation responses are effective; and they are used to make compounds called prostaglandins, which help with hormone regulation, cell growth, calcium mobilization, and pain reduction. But we need to eat these fatty acids in particular proportions or we increase the risk of imbalance. A healthy ratio of omega-6 fats to omega-3 fats is 1:1, or even up to about 4:1, yet most people eat these fats in a 20:1 ratio (other research shows that it might be closer to 40:1). A very high ratio of omega-6 to omega-3 fatty acids has been linked with cancer, inflammation, pain disorders, autoimmune diseases, and cardiovascular diseases—many of the same health problems associated with an overly acidic system.

THE MEAT OF THE MATTER

The average American eats 248 pounds of meat every year, about 40 percent of his or her total caloric intake. Our ancestors, in comparison, took in about 5 percent of their calories from animal protein (and, I might add, ate substantially less food overall than we do). Most experts agree that no more than 10 percent of our total calories should be obtained from meat.

We have already learned that the additives and preservatives used in meat are acidic. To further complicate things, meat itself is acid-forming in our bodies. Although research shows that meat tests alkaline before it is digested, once it mingles with the body's digestive juices and is metabolized, it leaves an acidic residue. As with any other acid-forming food, our bodies must try to neutralize and eliminate it.

Let's contrast the effects of meat and vegetables on our bodies to better understand the inherent problems with meat consumption. Vegetables typically have high concentrations of the minerals potassium, magnesium, and calcium. These foods break down into an alkaline ash that decreases acidity in the body. Diets high in meat, which is frequently combined with grains, are higher in iron, sulfur, and phosphorus. They create an acidic ash that acidifies our tissues and blood. These substances make our bodies work harder to keep our pH balanced so that our blood remains healthy. By drawing on alkaline substances from within our systems, the acid is neutralized. The more frequently we must do this, the greater the strain on our systems. We are, as the old adage states, robbing Peter to pay Paul. When our bodies can no longer keep up, we risk slipping into a state of pH imbalance, which we'll discuss further in the next chapter.

Some of the most acid-forming meats include beef, duck, chicken (and eggs), pork, and turkey. Seafood falls into this category as well. While all fish is acidic, farmed fish tends to be more acidic than wild fish. Don't worry: you don't have to give up meat entirely and become a strict vegetarian—unless, of course, you want to. While there is strong evidence of the health benefits of a vegetarian or largely vegetarian diet, your body is capable of overcoming the acidifying effects of minimal to moderate meat consumption.

FREQUENTLY ASKED QUESTIONS

Q: If I cut back on meat, how will I get adequate protein?

A: There is protein in every fruit, vegetable, grain, nut, bean, and seed. These foods also supply plentiful amounts of vitamins, minerals, fiber, phytochemicals (healing plant chemicals), enzymes, and beneficial fats. Most protein from non-meat sources is actually easier for the body to digest, extract, and use. A significant body of research—including the landmark China Study—indicates that we eat excessive amounts of protein, particularly from animal sources. In chapter 5, you'll learn about excellent vegetarian sources of protein.

GOT MILK?

The United States and Canada have two of the highest rates of dairy product consumption in the world. The average American drinks almost 18 gallons of milk and eats 12 pounds of cheese and 1.5 pounds of butter annually, while the typical Canadian drinks nearly 13 gallons of milk and eats 13 pounds of cheese and 3 pounds of butter every year. Yet levels of osteoporosis in North America are higher than ever and still climbing. By comparison, the diet of a typical Bantu woman in Africa is devoid of milk and other dairy products; her calcium intake comes solely from plant sources. Even though she obtains only half the average amount of calcium consumed by North American women, she is unlikely to ever suffer from osteoporosis: the disease is relatively unknown among Africans eating a traditional diet. Despite this evidence, North American government departments and dairy bureaus advise us that the way to counter osteoporosis and bone loss is to drink more milk.

Once consumed, dairy products contribute to acidity in multiple ways. They contain acidic saturated fats and acidic concentrated animal protein. And acidity plays a role in bone demineralization and osteoporosis, as you will discover in chapter 3.

WATER, WATER EVERYWHERE . . . AND NOT A DROP TO DRINK

Clean water is critical to life on this planet. Our health depends on it. Most people have heard that more than two-thirds of our body weight is water. Our blood is over 80 percent water. Our bones are 50 percent water. Every cell and organ requires water to function properly. Water helps to lubricate our joints, regulate metabolism, balance temperature, eliminate waste from our bodies, and ensure adequate electrical function so our brains and nervous systems function properly. Yet the vast majority of the population is dehydrated most of the time. When presented with alternatives like soda, coffee, lattes, and milk shakes, North Americans simply don't drink enough water on a daily basis.

Researchers estimate that 75 percent of Americans and half of the world's population are chronically dehydrated. That's a frightening statistic when you consider that many people worldwide suffer from dehydration because they live in developing nations without adequate access to drinking water. In the United States and Canada, where freshwater lakes and rivers abound and access to running water or well water is commonplace, there is little excuse for chronic dehydration. I am always astounded by the number of patients I see who drink only 1 or 2 cups of water a day, typically in the form of coffee. If you fall into this category, you'll likely see tremendous health improvements simply by increasing your water consumption. I will explain more about the health benefits of alkaline water in the coming chapters. For now, consider this: by increasing your water consumption to 5 cups per day (still an inadequate amount), you'll lower your risk of developing colon cancer by 45 percent, breast cancer by 79 percent, and bladder cancer by 50 percent.

Some people have a hard time accepting that something as simple as drinking more water is sufficient to make a difference to their health. Perhaps they believe they need potent synthetic chemicals, in the form of pharmaceutical drugs, to reduce uncomfortable symptoms. This way of thinking is truly outdated and demonstrates a lack of understanding about how the human body works. Research shows that increasing water consumption to 8 to 10 cups a day eases joint or back pain in 80 percent of sufferers. No drug even comes close to that level of effectiveness. And pure water causes no harmful side effects. Name one drug that can make that claim.

Over the course of an average day in a temperate climate, the human body loses approximately 2.6 quarts of water, through the lungs as water vapor, through the skin as sweat, or through the kidneys as urine. Some (a less significant amount in the absence of diarrhea) is also lost through the bowels. In a hot environment, or when exercising vigorously, we can easily lose several times this amount. Heavy exercise in high temperatures could cause the loss of over 2.6 quarts of fluid *per hour*, which exceeds the body's absorptive capacity. Even if we do absolutely nothing—we don't eat or drink, and we don't exercise—our bodies still lose about 1.3 quarts of water daily.

Our bodies need plentiful amounts of alkaline water. Yet most of our tap, bottled, and even purified water is acidic. There are thousands of possible pollutants in our water, and no testing is done for most of them. The U.S. Environmental Protection Agency lists only about 200 pollutants for which municipal and drinking water must be tested. Unfortunately, even these pollutants are not completely eliminated from our drinking water. Most of these chemicals contribute to the acidity of water, as does the addition of acidic chlorine and fluoride. Bottled water is not necessarily any better, as you will discover later.

THE COLA EXPERIMENT

Not only do most people not drink enough water, but they typically drink soda instead. That's a twofold insult to your body and your health. The average person guzzles 53 gallons of soda per year. That's about 848 cups, or almost 2½ cups per person per day. And you guessed it: carbonated beverages are extremely acidic. According to some research, the average can of Coca-Cola measures 2.52 on the pH scale.

Remember the tug-of-war analogy? Imagine that the rope measures from 0 to 14, with one team at the extremely acidic end, which is measured as 0, and the other team at the extremely alkaline end, which is measured as 14. Exactly in the middle, you'll find the neutral spot, or balance, which is measured as 7. Your body always strives for balance. The extremes of 0 or 14 would mean immediate death, and are never found in a living human body. Your body tries to maintain a tight balance between 6.8 (slightly acidic) and 7.4 (slightly alkaline).

Now that you've been primed on pH balance, it's clear that Coke's rating of 2.52 is extremely acidic! You're a Pepsi drinker? Studies have found that the average can of Pepsi measures 2.61, which is only marginally better. Surely Mountain Dew must contain some pure, alkaline mountain glacier water? No luck there either: it measures 3.27. Orange pop averages 2.90; Sprite averages 3.29; and root beer fares only slightly better at 4.24. No matter what type of soda you drink, you're giving your body a serious hit of acid. Researchers estimate that it takes 32 glasses of pure water with a pH reading of 7.0 to neutralize one glass of soda, diet or otherwise. That's clearly an impossible task for the average person over the course of an average day, even if one glass of soda were the only acidic food choice we had to compensate for.

A primary ingredient (other than acidic sugar or artificial sweeteners) in cola and other types of soda is phosphoric acid, which has a pH of 2.8—extremely acidic. Studies show that phosphoric acid leaches calcium and other minerals from bones, prevents mineral absorption, and contributes to osteoporosis.[6] Other research specifically links soda consumption to osteoporosis.[7]

Soda is a relatively new beverage. There are no rivers, lakes, and streams filled with this bubbly, acidic brew, and it is certainly not normal or healthy to be drinking it. Soda consumption, however, is not the only recent phenomenon causing us to experience disease in higher proportions than ever before.

BIGGIE-SIZING OURSELVES

What we eat is only part of the problem; as our food choices have changed over the years, our portion sizes have gradually increased. We have grown accustomed to "biggie-sizing" our meals, thanks to the campaigns of fast-food restaurants and the food processing industry. Even our so-called natural fruits, vegetables, and grains are getting bigger, through selective breeding, cultivation, and genetic modification. We've read or heard in the media that biggie-sizing is contributing to obesity. And indeed, obesity levels have skyrocketed over the past 20 years. But we don't need media reports to tell us that the human race is getting obese; all we have to do is look around us.

Recent data from the U.S. National Center for Health Statistics indicate that 30 percent of Americans 20 years or older are obese. That's 60 million adults. And another third of the population is overweight. In addition, the percentage of obese children has tripled since 1980. Information from the Centers for Disease Control and Prevention (CDC) states that more than 9 million children and teens between the ages of 6 and 19 are considered overweight. In Canada, according to Statistics Canada and the Treasury Board of Canada, the numbers are only slightly better: 23 percent of Canadian adults are obese, and 26.2 percent of children between the ages of 2 and 17 are overweight or obese.

While many people consider obesity a primarily North American phenomenon, the rates are climbing in Europe and Asia as well, including developing nations and, in some cases, regions that have suffered famine. On a global level, our relationship with food is clearly out of balance.

The repercussions of obesity extend far beyond simply being overweight. The CDC implicates obesity and overweight in many diseases and unhealthy conditions, including hypertension; dyslipidemia (high total cholesterol or high levels of triglycerides, for example); type 2 diabetes; coronary (heart) disease; stroke; gallbladder disease; osteoarthritis; sleep apnea and respiratory problems; and endometrial, breast, and colon cancers. Aside from the obvious suffering caused by obesity and the numerous diseases linked to it, the financial cost is huge. In the United States alone, obesity is responsible for $90 billion in medical costs and 300,000 premature deaths every year.

Health professionals use a measurement called body mass index (BMI), which takes both height and weight into account, to determine whether someone is overweight or obese. A BMI over 25 is considered overweight; a BMI over 30 is considered obese. Every day, another person steps into the overweight or obese category faster than you can say "double-glazed doughnut," and the trend shows no signs of reversing any time soon. If you haven't already watched Morgan Spurlock's entertaining and eye-opening documentary *Super Size Me*, I highly recommend that you do so (see the Resources on page 182 for more information).

It's clear that most of us consume high-fat, high-protein, high-sugar diets laden with food additives, added sodium, and trans or hydrogenated fats and consider our food choices completely normal. They may be common choices in our modern age of fast food, but they are not normal choices. The reality is that most people don't have a clue what a normal diet is, or should be. Obesity is bound to result when people eat a highly acidic diet: fat stores are your body's natural built-in protective mechanism against excessive acidity, which is potentially damaging to every cell in your body.

INDUSTRIALIZING OUR FOOD

There's a mountain of research that demonstrates the negative effects of fast food and processed, packaged, and prepared foods. Most researchers who study the effects of food industrialization on human health agree that our collective shift toward this type of highly acid-forming food is having significant health ramifications. Friedrich Manz, a professor and medical doctor with the Research Institute of Child Nutrition in Dortmund, Germany, has studied the history of nutrition and acid–base physiology. His work has illustrated the connection between acidic processed foods and nutritional deficiency disorders. He states: "In the industrializing countries, the preferred use of inexpensive non-perishable processed food products, such as superfine flour, resulted in epidemics of nutritional disorders at the beginning of the 20th century. In retrospect, the new epidemics were due to vitamin or trace element deficiencies or food intoxication."[8] Acidity is linked to both problems.

In another study that compared our acidity with that of our pre-agricultural ancestors, a team of scientists found that the nutrient composition of contemporary diets is completely misaligned with the genetically determined nutritional requirements for maintaining a healthy pH level: "In comparison with the diet habitually ingested by pre-agricultural *Homo sapiens* living in the Upper Paleolithic period (40,000–10,000 years ago), the diet of contemporary *Homo sapiens* (modern humans) is rich in saturated fat, simple sugars, sodium, and chloride and poor in fiber, magnesium, and potassium. These and numerous other post-agricultural dietary compositional changes have been implicated as risk factors in the pathogenesis of 'diseases of civilization,' including atherosclerosis, hypertension, type 2 diabetes, osteoporosis, and certain types of cancer."[9]

The researchers concluded that our pre-agricultural ancestors ate an alkaline-producing diet, based on alkaline plant foods. These healthy foods have been replaced in the contemporary diet by cereal grains (generally in the form of breads) and energy-dense (high-calorie), nutrient-poor foods—neither of which have alkaline-producing effects on our bodies. Consequently, our diets and our bodies are far more acidic and we suffer from diseases and disorders that could not take hold if we ate an alkalizing diet.

The introduction of farming—plants and animals—was one of the most profound technological advances and at the same time one of the worst dietary changes in human history. It increased human consumption of cereal grains and domesticated, fatty meats, while reducing our intake of a wide variety of wild plant species, many of which we would no longer recognize as food. Since then, we've degraded our food further with pesticides, antibiotics, synthetic hormones, and other unnatural chemicals, genetic modification, biochemical alterations, and more.

In his excellent book *Healing the Planet One Patient at a Time*, environmental medicine physician Dr. Jozef Krop asks, "When the food we eat is grown in nutrient-poor soil, watered with acid rain, sprayed with pesticides, and treated with food additives, and when the water we drink and the air we breathe are also contaminated, is it any wonder that chemicals have been detected in human blood and fat tissue?"[10] To that I would add, "Is it any wonder that we are suffering from so many chronic and life-threatening diseases?"

But we don't have to suffer needlessly. A life filled with health and vitality is yours for the taking. It is possible to have abundant energy, glowing skin, stable moods, balanced weight, and overall joie de vivre. I am excited to share with you what has taken me almost two decades of research to learn. Armed with this information, you can prevent and even reverse many health conditions by making simple changes to your food, beverage, and lifestyle choices. Stop suffering! In the coming pages, you'll learn the exciting secrets of great health and share in a revolutionary and natural approach to disease prevention and healing.

pH SOLUTION

Gordon Says Goodbye to Allergies

When I first met Gordon, he had a constantly runny nose from seasonal allergies. He carried tissues with him everywhere he went. When I examined him, I discovered that his body was highly acidic. I asked if he ate many sweets; to my surprise, he said he rarely did. But upon further questioning, I discovered that he regularly consumed sweetened "fruit juices," soda pop, sugary breakfast muffins, sugar-laden breads and buns, and many other hidden sugars. I believed that his consumption of sugar, dairy products, and large amounts of protein was creating an acid imbalance in his body.

I asked Gordon if he would be willing to eat an alkaline diet for two months, and he agreed to follow it faithfully. Each morning, he drank a large glass of purified water with half a lemon squeezed into it. He had never tried an avocado before, but when I told him they had a buttery taste and more usable protein than an 8-ounce steak, he was intrigued. Now avocado is one of his favorite foods. He switched from his favorite BLT to what he calls an ALT sandwich—avocado, lettuce, and tomato on sprouted grain bread. This is now his lunch of choice. He replaced cow's milk with almond milk as a base for smoothies, which he enjoys creating with his new high-powered blender. His wife loves his new interest in food and enjoys the many different smoothie recipes he whips up for their breakfast.

Even before he had completed the full two-month program, Gordon excitedly reported that he had lost his allergies! In fact, he had allowed himself to encounter many of his worst allergens, such as grasses and pollens, and had remained symptom-free. His nose had stopped running. His sneezing had stopped. His itchy eyes were clear, and his throat was no longer scratchy. "I feel like a free man!" he told me. He was able to pursue more outdoor activities, such as hiking and running, since he no longer suffered from the allergies that had held him back.

Gordon rigorously stuck to the program for two months; after that, he went back to occasionally eating some sugary foods, dairy products, and meat, but only in moderation. By sticking to the program in the beginning, he gave his body a chance to detoxify and strengthen. As long as he follows it fairly closely, his allergies are under control. If he feels his allergies start to creep back, he simply adds more alkalizing foods and stops eating sugar and dairy until he's feeling great again.

I was surprised when Gordon told me he had experienced a few side effects from his alkaline diet, but then he revealed with a grin what they were: his weight had stabilized, he was sleeping better than ever, he had lots more energy, and his mood swings were a thing of the past.

CHAPTER 2

Maintaining a Delicate Balance

"The best and safest thing is to keep a balance in your life, acknowledge the great powers around us and in us. If you can do that, and live that way, you are really a wise [wo]man."

—EURIPIDES

We've all heard about the ravages of acid rain. Resulting from toxic emissions in the environment, acid rain damages the leaves and needles on trees, reduces a tree's ability to withstand cold, drought, disease, and pests, and even inhibits or prevents plant reproduction. In an effort to stay alive and combat the acidity, tree roots pull important nutrients such as calcium and magnesium from the soil. These alkaline nutrients balance the effects of acid rain, but as they become depleted from the soil, the trees' ability to survive is further strained.

The average pH of rain in the eastern American states and in southern Ontario and Quebec is about 40 times more acidic than experts suggest it should be. That water acidifies soil, lakes, and the air, over time causing significant and potentially irreversible damage to the whole ecosystem.[1] In addition, higher acidity in seawater reduces the oxygen available to marine creatures and prevents the proper formation of skeletons. This means a reduction in the food supply for both marine life and humans.

A highly acidic diet is like acid rain in our bloodstreams. We are polluting our bodies on an individual level the same way we are polluting our planet. Because of our poor choices, we are essentially microcosms of the same problems our planet faces. The difference is that most of us are aware that we are polluting the planet, yet few of us realize that we are subjecting our bodies to similar internal pollution and acid waste.

Like trees and sea creatures, to support our internal habitat we need water that is neither too acidic nor too alkaline. In the United States, over 80 percent

23

of the population gets its water from community water supplies. Private water sources and wells supply the rest. But all types of water systems are susceptible to pollution and contaminants from diverse sources, such as pesticides and fertilizers, petroleum products, viruses, bacteria, and algae. The pH balance of drinking water can also be compromised by natural geological conditions and acid rain (this is particularly true for well water or surface water); chemicals added at water treatment facilities; corrosion from plumbing; and leaching of metals, such as copper, lead, iron, cadmium, and zinc, into the water supply. (To learn more about the dangers of heavy metals and toxins to the brain and nervous system, read my book *The Brain Wash*.)

In addition to clean water, we (like trees and sea creatures) need an oxygenated environment in our bodies. If we lack oxygen at the cellular level, we create an environment that is ripe for anaerobic (meaning "without oxygen") fermentation, the type of environment in which yeasts, fungi, molds, and cancers thrive. (I will discuss this further in chapter 3.)

Throughout this chapter, you will learn more about what pH is; what acidity and alkalinity are; why it is likely that your body is acidic; why you need to prevent your body from becoming acidic, or bring it back into balance if it already is acidic; and the benefits of maintaining a balanced pH throughout your life. Armed with this knowledge, you will be able to prevent acidity from damaging your body and making you more susceptible to disease.

ACID–ALKALINE BALANCE 101

If you've ever tried cleaning your home with vinegar and baking soda, you already know about pH, perhaps without even realizing it. Vinegar is acidic and baking soda is alkaline. When you mix the two together, they fizz and fizzle and neutralize each other.

The term "pH" (pronounced just like the letters "p-h") stands for "potential of hydrogen," which is the measure of any solution's hydrogen ion concentration. It's not necessary to delve into hydrogen ions to grasp this topic; I'll leave that to the biochemists. As you learned in the previous chapter, pH is a measure of acidity or alkalinity on a scale of 0 to 14. Zero is extremely acidic, while 14 is extremely alkaline (or basic, as it is also known). In the middle, at 7, the pH is neutral, meaning there is complete balance between acid and base.

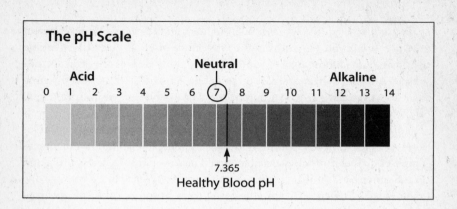

Our blood and most of our tissues need to remain balanced in the neutral to slightly alkaline zone for optimum health. Our bowels should be slightly acidic. Urine needs to be between neutral and slightly acidic. Saliva tends to fluctuate more between acid, alkaline, and neutral. But overall, keeping your blood slightly alkaline is the primary goal, since blood nourishes your tissues, organs, and organ systems. This acid–base balancing act occurs within a very small range at the cellular level. Every single cell has a small optimum range within which it performs its many functions. Different cell types have different ranges, but regardless of the range, the pH of our bodies is tightly controlled near the middle of the scale.

The Standard American Diet and the stressful lifestyle most of us follow tip the scale in favor of acidity, creating an imbalance and forcing our bodies to deal with a continual—or chronic—state of acidity at the metabolic level. It is not so severe that you would be hospitalized because your body is acidic. That condition, known as metabolic acidosis, does occur but is usually associated with a pre-existing disease. We won't be delving into this severe disorder in *The Ultimate pH Solution*, but will instead focus on smaller, more gradual changes and the effects they have on our health, our sense of well-being, and our vulnerability to disease over time.

The Perfect Balance

Ideally, your blood needs to be maintained around pH 7.365, which is slightly alkaline. A change from pH 7.0 to pH 6.0 indicates a *tenfold* increase in acidity, since each point along the spectrum is measured to one decimal place. In other words, as your saliva pH drops from 7.0 (acidic) to 6.0 (even more acidic), it first drops to 6.9, then 6.8, then 6.7, and so on until it reaches 6.0, at which point you have 10 times more acidity in your body. Even worse than that, in the blood, it takes approximately 20 times as much of an alkaline substance to neutralize one part of an acidic substance! That's why it takes so many cups of water to neutralize one cup of cola, as you learned in the previous chapter.

You don't want the balance in your body to swing too far in either direction—either acid or base—since both have potentially harmful health effects. If your body is chronically too acidic, you'll be susceptible to health problems; on the other hand, if it is chronically too alkaline, you're likely to have different health problems. So why do I refer to this program as Kick Acid, not Kick Acid and Base? Well, most people's bodies lean toward acidic, and many people's bodies are extremely acidic, making them vulnerable to a whole host of illnesses. Very few people have an alkaline, or basic, pH. Those who do are typically extremely acidic. That might sound confusing and contradictory, but bear with me while I explain how the body tries to keep acid under control.

Acidic foods such as burgers, fries, steak, milk, cake, candy, and soda pop tip the balance toward the acid side. To counter this acid onslaught, your body releases alkaline substances from your organs, bones, and tissues. A measurement taken at this time may reveal an alkaline pH because your body has just dumped minerals from your tissues to counter excessive acidity. Your body knows that if your blood becomes too acidic you will die. (Actually, the human body becomes acidic upon death, but that's another story.)

It is rare to find someone who actually is too alkaline on an ongoing basis. Such a person would likely eat a vegan diet (vegetarian with no dairy, eggs, or other animal products), avoiding all fast food, processed food, packaged food, fruit, and sweets. Even then, it is rather unlikely. So even if you never test your pH (although I encourage you to give it a try, since it tends to be eye-opening), your diet is almost certainly too acidic. Keep in mind that an absence of symptoms does not mean that your body is in balance.

Acidic Blood

Throughout this book, we will be discussing what happens when your blood deals with excessive amounts of acid from your diet and lifestyle choices. I will be referring to this situation as acidic blood. Please remember that your blood never truly becomes acidic by medical standards. You would die long before that ever happened. Your body keeps regulating and responding to situations that increase the level of acidity in your system to ensure that your blood maintains that very narrow, slightly alkaline range required for healthy function.

However, the foods we eat, the liquids we drink, the substances to which we are exposed, shallow breathing, and lack of exercise do have the potential to increase acidity in our body and negatively affect our blood. This happens because our body stores excess acid in our tissues, causing a decrease in their pH. Our blood tries to compensate by pulling from stores in our body to become slightly more alkaline.

If our blood's pH is constantly unbalanced, even a little bit, it is no longer effective at neutralizing and eliminating acid waste products from our systems. The more they build up and the longer they persist, the more likely that disease will take hold.

TESTING YOUR BODY'S pH LEVEL

There are various tests that can help you determine whether your body is acidic, including saliva, urine, and blood tests. While some manufacturers claim that saliva and urine tests are equally effective, urine testing is actually more accurate. But it is important to do whatever you are most comfortable with. If the thought of testing your urine makes you squeamish, test your saliva. You're not looking for exact measurements here. Instead, you want to find out approximately how acid or alkaline you are, particularly watching for any trends over time.

Saliva Testing

Saliva testing gives a general range of the saliva's pH and should be used only as a rough guide. Over time, it can provide a broad picture of a person's overall state of acid–alkaline balance.

Saliva testing is easy and inexpensive. Simply buy some pH paper, which comes in a small roll and is available at most health food stores. It usually costs between $10 and $15.

The color coding system tends to vary from one brand to another, but the process is the same. Simply tear off a 1- to 2-inch strip and place it under your tongue in some saliva. Try not to let it touch your tongue, lips, or gums. Immediately check the strip's color against the color scale on the back of the roll. Use this immediate reading, as the strip changes color as the paper dries. You'll usually get a reading between 6.0 (acidic) and 8.0 (alkaline), although some people may test lower than 6.0.

The best time to test your saliva is first thing in the morning, before you eat or drink anything. You'll get a more accurate idea of your body's pH level if, over time, you keep a log of the first test of the morning and watch for trends. If your pH level routinely tests acidic but you have an occasional alkaline reading, you are likely quite acidic; your body may be dumping alkaline minerals from your muscles, bones, or organs to compensate.

Urine Testing

Urine testing also uses pH paper. It is more accurate than saliva testing, but should still be used only as a general guideline. To test your urine, place a 2-inch or longer strip of pH paper in the urine stream. If that is too difficult, collect some of your urine in a paper cup and dip one side of the pH paper strip into it. As with saliva testing, this is best done first thing in the morning, any time after 4:00 a.m., when you first urinate after awakening. Immediately compare the color of the pH paper to the color scale on the back of the roll. Keep a log of your results over time and watch for trends indicative of acidity. Urine usually tests slightly more acidic than saliva, which is to be expected.

Blood Testing

Blood testing is the most accurate way to evaluate your pH level, but gives you only a snapshot of your blood's acid–alkaline balance at a particular time on a particular day, which is of little value when you're trying to determine whether your blood pH levels show a trend toward acidity. Because blood testing is conducted by your medical doctor and the tests are sent to a laboratory for results, it is less convenient and more expensive than other forms of testing.

Interpreting Your Readings

When I was conducting research for this book, I became alarmed at the amount of misinformation out there. Websites contradict each other. Health food store brochures and magazine articles dole out completely inaccurate information. Even "experts," companies that manufacture pH products, and book authors give contradictory advice. So I'm never surprised when people express frustration and confusion about interpreting their pH readings.

Forget what you've read elsewhere. I've sifted through the volumes of data for you, eliminating the inaccuracies and paring the information down to the essentials. Ideally, your saliva pH should be between 7.0 and 7.4, while your urine pH should be around 6.8.

If you sometimes test acidic and other times quite alkaline, you may wonder what's going on in your body. Remember that your body uses built-in mechanisms to restore balance. If you primarily test acidic (for example, 6.2) and occasionally test alkaline (for example, 8.0), that typically means that your body is dumping minerals from your bones or muscles to compensate for acidity. In other words, even when you test alkaline, it is often a sign of acidity. If you always seem to test alkaline, particularly highly alkaline (around 8.0), it is usually a sign that your body is consistently dumping minerals from your bones or muscles to nullify excessive acidity.

FREQUENTLY ASKED QUESTIONS

Q: Do I need to test my pH to benefit from the Kick Acid program?

A: No. Even if you are extremely health-conscious, it's likely that you are eating an acidic diet. It is safe to assume that you are acidic and follow the Kick Acid program. Because the program emphasizes balance and healing, you will benefit from the program whether you are too acidic or, in the rarest of situations, too alkaline.

Testing your pH provides you with information for a particular point in time. Many people are motivated by visible, tangible evidence, and testing your pH provides that evidence. But some people are very good at measuring results by how they feel. After eating an alkaline diet for a few days, you may realize that your energy level has increased, you are not as bloated, and you no longer have heartburn. You may be sleeping better, and symptoms such as pain, allergies, and infections may be improving.

The goal of the Kick Acid program is to introduce you to delicious low-acid, high-alkaline food options that, combined with simple lifestyle changes, take the acid strain off your body. When your body has more energy to conduct its normal functions, instead of fighting to balance your acid load, you have more energy for healing and living life to the fullest. Plus, you ward off disease and illness in the process.

WHAT CAUSES ACIDITY IN THE BODY?

There are many factors that contribute to acid buildup in the body, including stress, toxins, infections, and an acidic diet.

Stress

Let's face it, most of us are dealing with high levels of chronic stress. Stress has become a way of life for many people. Some even brag about how much stress they're handling, how overworked they are, or how many hours a day they work. Others seek out added stress by undertaking extreme sports in an attempt to get the next adrenaline rush.

Regardless of the type of stress you are facing, your body pumps out hormones to help you deal with it. But your body doesn't differentiate between chronic job stress and more primitive types of stress such as running from a wild animal. So these hormones help send blood to your limbs even at the expense of your brain and quicken your breathing to help you run or fight—whichever you choose to do—what we know as "fight or flight." That might work if you're facing a tiger, but it doesn't help with chronic job or home stresses, where clear thinking would serve you better than fighting with your boss or running away from your screaming children.

While these hormones definitely have their place, they effectively acidify your body if they are chronically secreted by your glands. In addition, because chronic stress causes us to either breathe faster (not deeper) or hold our breath, we are prone to more acidity. That's because our oxygen intake drops, and oxygen alkalizes our blood, as well as all of the tissues and organs the blood nourishes.

Toxins

You learned a bit about the toxins found in our food in the previous chapter, but we are exposed to many more toxins than that. There are more than 80,000 industrial chemicals in use today, many of which find their way into our air, water, or food. While there are some naturally formed toxins in our air and water, the majority are the result of industrial emissions or dumping. In 2000, more than 4 billion pounds of chemicals were released into the ground and almost 2 billion pounds of chemical emissions were pumped into the atmosphere. The National Research Council in Canada has no toxicity data on over

80 percent of the chemicals in commercial use, primarily because most of have not been studied for their effects on humans. Many of these toxins find t way into our bodies through the air we breathe or through our drinking water.

Plentiful amounts of toxins are also found in our laundry detergents, fabric softeners (don't be fooled by their lovely names and pretty scents—these chemicals are some of the worst health offenders), room deodorizers, perfumes, colognes, air fresheners, cosmetics, and personal hygiene products. For eye-opening information on the effects of these toxins, the many hidden places they lurk, and how to eliminate them from your body, read my books *The Brain Wash* and *The 4-Week Ultimate Body Detox Plan*. Regardless of how you come into contact with them, the majority of these toxins acidify your body.

Infections

We are exposed to thousands of different types of bacteria, viruses, fungi, yeasts, molds, amoebas, and other microbes on a regular basis. Many of these germs live within our bodies. An acidic body is the perfect environment for them to survive and thrive. Worse, once germs take up residence in our bodies, the by-products of their metabolism are also acidic. According to many experts, the over-acidification of our bodily fluids and tissues is the precursor to microbial infections. Only when a body is acidic will it be vulnerable to germs. When our bodies lean toward a slightly alkaline state, germs cannot survive.

People regularly blame their cold or flu virus on someone who "gave" it to them at a party during the holiday season, but an examination of the type of diet we eat during the holidays holds more clues as to where that infection originated. Just a few tablespoons of sugar in a yummy dessert can depress your immune system for four to six hours, giving germs a chance to take hold in your body. By then, you may be craving the next sweet dessert, thanks to blood sugar fluctuations caused by the first. What's the likelihood that you overindulged in acidic sweets or other acidic foods during the holidays? Considering that acidic foods make up the bulk of our diet, the odds are very good indeed.

Acidic Diet

An acid-forming diet is potentially the worst culprit in affecting our pH balance. Sweets, meat, dairy, trans fats, chemical additives, white flour, fried foods, and many other acidic foods can make it difficult for our bodies to restore balance.

c acid load on our glands, organs, tissues, and blood can
percussions. To worsen the situation, acidic foods lack
minerals, fiber, enzymes, and other nutritional compo-
lies restore balance, which adds further strain to our
wielmed systems. We'll discuss which acidic foods to reduce or
eliminate from your diet, as well as which ones are worth keeping, in chapter 4.

HOW WELL DO YOU KICK ACID?

It's time for a little eye-opening fun. Grab a pencil and paper to keep track of your points—and be honest!

Section A: Diet and Lifestyle

1. I add sugar or artificial sweeteners to tea, coffee, cereal, or other food or drinks
    - 2 or more times a day (5 points)
    - Once a day (4 points)
    - 3 to 6 times a week (3 points)
    - Once or twice a week (2 points)
    - Less than once a week (1 point)
    - Never (0 points)

2. I eat fried foods (including battered chicken and fish, french fries, pre-fried packaged foods, etc.)
    - 2 or more times a day (5 points)
    - Once a day (4 points)
    - 3 to 6 times a week (3 points)
    - Once or twice a week (2 points)
    - Less than once a week (1 point)
    - Never (0 points)

3. I eat desserts (cake, cookies, doughnuts, pies, etc.) and drink sweetened drinks (including sport drinks, iced tea, lemonade, and bottled fruit juices)
    - 2 or more times a day (5 points)
    - Once a day (4 points)
    - 3 to 6 times a week (3 points)
    - Once or twice a week (2 points)
    - Less than once a week (1 point)
    - Never (0 points)

4. I drink cola or other soda (any kind, regular or diet)
- 2 or more times a day (6 points)
- Once a day (5 points)
- 3 to 6 times a week (4 points)
- Once or twice a week (3 points)
- Less than once a week (2 points)
- Never (0 points)

5. I eat fast food (burgers, fries, onion rings, tacos, pizza, subs, etc.)
- 2 or more times a day (5 points)
- Once a day (4 points)
- 3 to 6 times a week (3 points)
- Once or twice a week (2 points)
- Less than once a week (1 point)
- Never (0 points)

6. I eat convenience store snacks (chocolate bars, chips, Slurpees, etc.)
- 2 or more times a day (5 points)
- Once a day (4 points)
- 3 to 6 times a week (3 points)
- Once or twice a week (2 points)
- Less than once a week (1 point)
- Never (0 points)

7. I eat or drink dairy products (milk, cheese, ice cream, yogurt, etc.)
- 2 or more times a day (4 points)
- Once a day (3 points)
- 3 to 6 times a week (2 points)
- Once or twice a week (1 point)
- Less than once a week (1 point)
- Never (0 points)

8. I eat processed, packaged foods (boxed cereals, microwaveable meals, canned soups and sauces, TV dinners, etc.)
- 2 or more times a day (5 points)
- Once a day (4 points)
- 3 to 6 times a week (3 points)
- Once or twice a week (2 points)
- Less than once a week (1 point)
- Never (0 points)

9. I eat red meat and/or pork
- 2 or more times a day (5 points)
- Once a day (4 points)

- 3 to 6 times a week (3 points)
- Once or twice a week (2 points)
- Less than once a week (1 point)
- Never (0 points)

10. I eat chicken and/or fish (not fried or battered)
- 2 or more times a day (4 points)
- Once a day (3 points)
- 3 to 6 times a week (2 points)
- Once or twice a week (1 point)
- Less than once a week (1 point)
- Never (0 points)

11. I smoke cigarettes
- 2 or more times a day (5 points)
- Once a day (4 points)
- 3 to 6 times a week (3 points)
- Once or twice a week (2 points)
- Less than once a week (1 point)
- Never (0 points)

12. I drink alcohol (a glass of wine, beer, or other alcoholic beverage)
- 2 or more times a day (5 points)
- Once a day (4 points)
- 3 to 6 times a week (3 points)
- Once or twice a week (2 points)
- Less than once a week (1 point)
- Never (0 points)

13. I take over-the-counter or prescription medications
- 2 or more times a day, or more than one medication (5 points)
- Once a day (4 points)
- 3 to 6 times a week (3 points)
- Once or twice a week (2 points)
- Less than once a week (1 point)
- Never (0 points)

14. I feel stressed about my life/job/relationship
- 2 or more times a day (5 points)
- Once a day (4 points)
- 3 to 6 times a week (3 points)
- Once or twice a week (2 points)
- Less than once a week (1 point)
- Never (0 points)

15. I use personal care products and household cleaning products other than those sold in reputable health food stores.
- 2 or more times a day (3 points)
- Once a day (2 points)
- 3 to 6 times a week (2 points)
- Once or twice a week (1 point)
- Less than once a week (1 point)
- Never (0 points)

16. I eat pastries, breads, cereals, or baked goods containing white flour.
- 2 or more times a day (5 points)
- Once a day (4 points)
- 3 to 6 times a week (3 points)
- Once or twice a week (2 points)
- Less than once a week (1 point)
- Never (0 points)

SECTION A TOTAL: _____

Section B: Symptoms and Disease

Give yourself 3 points for every symptom or illness below that you experience on an ongoing basis (daily) and any disease or disorder you have been diagnosed with; 2 points for every symptom or illness you experience commonly (weekly); 1 point for every symptom or illness you experience infrequently (1 to 2 times a year); and 0 points if you don't experience the symptom or illness at all. Count only one symptom or illness per line. For example, if you experience both asthma and allergies on an ongoing basis, you would give yourself 3 points for that line. If you experience allergies on an ongoing basis and asthma weekly, you would still count 3 points for that line.

- Allergies, asthma, other respiratory concerns
- Arteriosclerosis, heart disease, heart attack, stroke, high cholesterol
- Arthritis, gout, ankylosing spondylitis
- Alzheimer's disease, Parkinson's disease, senility, dementia, other brain disorders
- Bronchitis, tonsillitis, laryngitis, other respiratory infections
- Cancer
- Chronic fatigue syndrome (diagnosed), fibromyalgia, environmental illness
- Colds or flu (more than once a year)
- Depression
- Diabetes
- Digestive concerns: pain, indigestion, constipation, diarrhea, heartburn, irritable bowel syndrome, colitis
- Gynecological problems: yeast infection, endometriosis, premenstrual syndrome, menopausal symptoms

- Headaches or migraines
- Hormonal imbalances
- Kidney disease or urinary tract infections
- Muscle loss, cramping, or wasting
- Multiple sclerosis, muscular dystrophy
- Osteoporosis, bone density loss, fractures or bone breaks
- Pain or discomfort
- Premature aging or graying
- Prostate problems
- Sinusitis or rhinitis
- Tooth decay, loss of teeth
- Weight gain, obesity, difficulty losing weight, difficulty gaining weight

SECTION B TOTAL: _____

COMBINED SECTION A + SECTION B TOTAL: _____

Section C: Healthy Living

I suspect most people are horrified and dismayed when they tally up their scores. I'm going to give you a chance to improve them without cheating. Simply calculate your score for the questions below:

1. I eat cooked or raw vegetables
   - 4 or more times a day (4 points)
   - 2 or 3 times a day (2 points)
   - Once a day (1 point)
   - Less than once a day (0 points)

2. I drink filtered water or alkaline water
   - 10 cups or more a day (4 points)
   - 7 to 9 cups a day (2 points)
   - 4 to 7 cups a day (1 point)
   - Less than 4 cups a day (0 points)

3. I exercise for at least 30 minutes (including walking at least 10,000 steps)
   - Every day (4 points)
   - 4 to 6 times a week (3 points)
   - 2 to 3 times a week (2 points)
   - Once a week (1 point)
   - Less than once a week (0 points)

4. I take time for myself (meditation, rest, relaxation of at least 30 minutes)
   - Every day (4 points)
   - 4 to 6 times a week (3 points)

- 2 to 3 times a week (2 points)
- Once a week (1 point)
- Less than once a week (0 points)

SECTION C TOTAL: _____

After you total your score for the questions in Section C, subtract this number from your original score (A + B) above. Did it change your rank?

FINAL TOTAL (A + B – C): _____

Final Scores

- **Over 50:** Danger zone. Your body is dealing with chronic high levels of acidity and will rarely have a balanced pH unless it robs your bones, tissues, and organs of existing stores of alkaline substances. Your health is in danger, assuming that you have not already been diagnosed with a major illness. The time for change is now. It's not too late to balance your body chemistry and start reaping the rewards. Read on!
- **35 to 50:** Warning alarms are sounding. Your diet and lifestyle are too acidic. You may already be experiencing symptoms of an unbalanced pH, such as fatigue, infections, inflammation, digestive problems, and allergies. You are eating the textbook Standard American Diet. You need to address diet and lifestyle issues to decrease your exposure to acidic foods and habits. *The Ultimate pH Solution* will show you how.
- **20 to 35:** You probably feel you live a fairly healthy lifestyle. Compared to most North Americans, you do. But your diet is still too acidic, and you may be paying a high price for your choices, even if you haven't started to experience symptoms yet. Read on to learn how to make your "healthy lifestyle" truly healthy.
- **10 to 20:** You are well on your way toward balancing your biochemistry. Sure, you have moments of weakness, but overall you are giving your body a fighting chance to maintain a slightly alkaline condition. If all your points came from one or two areas, you already know what you need to do. *The Ultimate pH Solution* will help you fine-tune your lifestyle for optimum health for life.
- **Under 10:** This is the pH equivalent of Mensa. Very few people will find themselves in this range. If your score is this low, congratulations. Share your successes with your friends and family and support them as they try to reduce their acidity. You will still benefit from reading *The Ultimate pH Solution*, as it will teach you how to tip the pH scales back into balance for those times when you're too acidic.

WHAT ARE THE EFFECTS OF CHRONIC ACIDITY?

Traditional research into human physiology suggests that because healthy humans have built-in mechanisms that maintain blood pH within a very narrow range, acidity will not cause problems. The kidneys, for example, are detoxification organs designed to excrete acid to help us keep the balance (or homeostasis) required for the proper functioning of our cells and systems. Consequently, many physiologists and researchers believed that our increasingly acidic diet could not alter blood pH in any measurable way. They continue to believe that the body always keeps the blood in a tight balance at 7.365 pH and that acid–alkaline balance doesn't stray far one way or another. The same people suggest that eating an acid-forming diet has no effect on blood or tissue pH because the body always restores balance.

I agree with the traditional medical belief that the body always works to restore balance. The familiar concept of body temperature provides a useful example. The human body needs to maintain a fairly tight temperature range, ideally around 98.6°F. Anything much lower than that and we start shivering in an effort to increase body temperature. Anything much higher and we run a fever, which causes us to start sweating in an effort to reduce body temperature.

Your body is constantly striving for a healthy biochemical balance as well. It tries to maintain homeostasis through many different means, including breathing, blood circulation, digestion, and hormone production. In addition to these basic life functions, the body has intrinsic ways of restoring pH balance when it is shifting too far to the acid side of the spectrum: it excretes toxic acids from the blood via the kidneys, and it dumps alkaline minerals from other locations in the body into the blood to neutralize the acidity.

However, recent research shows that our modern diet, full of acid-forming foods, *is* disrupting our acid–base metabolism. The body's acid-controlling mechanisms were intended to handle minor variations in pH; they were not designed to balance the effects of regular consumption of soda, huge quantities of meat, and high amounts of sugar, food additives, and fake and unhealthy fats. Nor were they designed to cope with the strain of a chronically stressful life. As a result, these mechanisms are extremely overtaxed.

The constant battle waged by your cells and organs to regulate your body's pH can take its toll, leading to health problems and disease. Disease can be either the direct result of acidity or the result of your body's inability to keep up with the acid load it faces, which leads to taxed organs and systems and depleted mineral reserves.

Symptoms and Chronic Illnesses

Common early signs of an acid–alkaline imbalance include headaches, pain, allergies, skin troubles, susceptibility to cold and flu viruses, sinus problems, breathing disorders, fatigue, inflammation, indigestion, and muscle cramping. These symptoms, and many others, are linked to an acid imbalance in your body, even if a doctor has told you that there are other factors involved.

Over time, your symptoms can worsen as your organs and glands start to be affected. Some of the first organs to succumb include the thyroid glands, the adrenal glands, and the liver. When your pH becomes chronically acidic, oxygen levels decrease and cells can die. Any number of chronic illnesses, ranging from asthma and allergies to arthritis or cancer, can form. You'll learn more about the acid–disease connection in chapter 3.

Acidity and Enzymes

An acidic diet can cause further damage by reducing enzymes in the body. Enzymes are critical to our health, and their significance is often overlooked. These proteins consist of long chains of amino acids. The specific sequence of the amino acids creates a unique enzyme structure with a specific purpose. Enzymes are needed for virtually every cell process, including metabolism, and they act as catalysts for more than 4,000 biochemical reactions required to keep us healthy.

Enzymes are found within our bodies, as well as in the food we eat. While they serve a multitude of functions, their role in the digestive system is what is important here. Certain enzymes break down larger molecules of protein and starch so that they can be effectively absorbed by the intestines. Proper metabolism is dependent on enzymes and coenzymes (molecules that transport chemicals from enzyme to enzyme). Often these chemicals cannot be manufactured in the body and are obtained through the food we eat . . . assuming we eat food that contains them!

Fruits and vegetables are our primary source of enzymes. However, enzymes are temperature-sensitive, and heat can damage or destroy them. Cooking fruits or vegetables at temperatures above 118°F, for example, renders the enzymes useless to our bodies. We still benefit from the non–heat-sensitive nutrients and compounds in the produce, but we force our digestive system to work harder with fewer resources.

Enzyme activity is also affected by pH. The more acidic we are, the less effective our enzyme activity. This has an impact on our digestion and most other bodily functions. In addition, enzyme function can be inhibited by drugs and toxins, which further interfere with bodily processes, increasing the likelihood of an acid–base imbalance. And, when the body uses minerals such as calcium and magnesium to nullify excessive acid, there may be inadequate amounts of these minerals available to jump-start enzyme processes—one of many important functions these minerals serve. If enzymes can't play their proper role, we become vulnerable to any number of possible illnesses.

WHAT DO WE MEAN BY METABOLISM?

Metabolism is the process of converting the food we ingest into the energy we require to run our body systems and functions. This is a biochemical process that feeds our cells and keeps us alive. Metabolism has two distinct parts: anabolism and catabolism. Anabolism refers to the cells' use of energy to perform life functions, such as building complex molecules and cell structure. Catabolism refers to the breakdown of complex molecules to release energy.

Metabolism is a complex reaction that creates heat, carbon dioxide, water, and waste. Much of the waste produced comes from acidic food that we ingested. The old computer science aphorism GIGO (garbage in, garbage out) is relevant to metabolism. If we ingest processed, chemical-laden, additive-filled food, our body cannot metabolize it properly and it creates an abundance of acidic waste. Somehow, we must find a way to remove this acid before it does damage.

Mineral Assimilation

Chronic acidity can also interfere with the body's ability to use the minerals in our diets for their respective functions. Some minerals require a fairly narrow pH range for proper assimilation. Iodine, which is linked with proper thyroid function, needs an almost ideal pH balance to be useful to our thyroid. Calcium and potassium can be assimilated in a relatively wide pH range, and sodium and magnesium have an even greater range. Assimilation ranges for zinc, copper, iron, and manganese fall between those of iodine and calcium. Even one mineral deficiency caused by excess acidity can throw off a range of body functions and lead to serious health concerns.

The Effects of Aging

As we age, our systems tend to become less effective due to the wear and tear of modern life. Our detoxification organs, our muscles, and our bones may weaken as time passes, and their capacity to deal with acidity can become compromised. Unfortunately, many people choose a diet and lifestyle that accelerate this wear and tear, resulting in more serious health conditions at an earlier age. By placing a greater burden on the body systems that cope with pH balance, we increase the risk of many diseases that have been linked with high metabolic acid creation in the body, including gout, osteoporosis, cystic fibrosis, thyroid problems, fibromyalgia, irritable bowel syndrome, cancer, and many other diseases, some of which we'll explore in detail in chapter 3. I would not be surprised to learn that the bone loss and muscle wasting associated with old age are in part due to—and worsened by—our addiction to highly acidic diets, or that age-related health problems such as osteoporosis could be minimized by smarter nutritional choices.

HOW DO OUR BODIES EXPEL AND NEUTRALIZE ACID?

A healthy human body maintains a proper acid–alkaline balance primarily by doing two things: expelling excess acid through the detoxification organs and neutralizing acid with alkaline substances, such as calcium or magnesium, that have been stored in the body and are derived from dietary sources.

Expelling Acid

Typically, your body tries to eliminate excess acid before it resorts to neutralizing the acid that's left over. The kidneys are the frontline soldiers in the body's war on acid, expelling acid as quickly as possible in the form of urine. Other key players are the lungs and the lymphatic system.

The Kidneys
The kidneys are two small, oval organs located on the left and right sides of the back at about the same level as the lower ribs, which partially cover and protect the kidneys. They have several key functions: they filter blood but also provide it with the good sugars, water, and amino acids required for healthy bodily function; they strive to maintain balance in your body, particularly fluid,

mineral, and pH balance; they excrete toxins (including excess acidity); and they regulate blood pressure through hormone production. They do all this for us, yet we rarely give these crucial detoxification organs a second thought unless we develop some form of kidney disorder.

The kidneys attempt to excrete, via the urine, toxins that have found their way into the blood. Toxins can enter the body from the air we breathe, the food we eat, or the beverages we drink. Toxins can also be created within the body as the by-products of normal metabolism or as a result of excess stress hormones linked to a chronically stressful life. Toxins may also be the by-products of viruses, bacteria, fungi, or other pathogens that inhabit our bodies (more on this topic later).

Regardless of where toxins originate, they have two things in common: (1) they can clog natural processes in the body, so they need to be filtered from the blood, and (2) the vast majority of them are acidic and, if allowed to stay in the body, could cause a buildup of acidity. So while there are many other organs and organ systems that detoxify the body, the kidneys play a doubly important role in balancing pH.

The kidneys must eliminate acid waste products when high-protein foods are broken down into their key components, called amino acids. Amino acids are essential to your body's health and are used to build healthy tissue. However, urea, an acidic by-product of protein metabolism, can build up in the body if you are eating too much protein for your kidneys to handle. While they are common, high-animal-protein diets are merely fad diets that result in overburdened kidneys and excess acid buildup.

If the kidneys cannot function properly because of excess urea and are thus unable to remove acids and toxins from the blood, these acids and toxins may be deposited in your tissues, resulting in pain, inflammation, or weight gain. There are three simple ways to help your kidneys detoxify acid wastes:

- Eat less acid-forming food (you'll learn how to do this in chapter 4).
- Eat more alkaline-forming food (you'll learn how to do this in chapter 5).
- Drink more pure, alkaline water to help the kidneys flush toxins.

To learn more about detoxifying the kidneys, consult my book *The 4-Week Ultimate Body Detox Plan*.

Let's briefly revisit the Standard American Diet on a more personal level to learn what happens when you eat a hamburger. As you chow down on that burger, you are ingesting everything on it to help fuel and build your body and mind. You're ingesting the white flour bun, the grilled meat, the lettuce, tomato, and onion. You're ingesting the sugary ketchup, the artificially colored mustard, and that pile of goop called relish that barely resembles food anymore. You're also ingesting all the chemicals, additives, and preservatives that found their way into the burger, bun, and toppings as these foods were raised or grown and processed.

All these nutrients, chemicals, and toxins are absorbed and ultimately find their way to the kidneys as an acid-forming compound or an alkaline-forming compound. In this case, the burger meal is almost exclusively acidic, so the kidneys have substantial work cut out for them.

More acidic compounds than alkaline ones create a net acid load on your body. I'm not talking about heartburn here, although you may experience that as well. Net acid load in this case means that the acidity of the hamburger meat, bun, and condiments outweighs any alkaline-producing micronutrients found in the vegetable slices and leafy greens and creates an acidic state in our bodies. We perpetuate this acid imbalance meal after meal by eating the Standard American Diet and ultimately increase the risk of long-term health problems and serious disease by straining our already overworked kidneys.

When our blood is acidic, the kidneys excrete ammonia into our urine, so strong-smelling urine can be a clue that our body is becoming acidic. Urinary infections may also be a sign of excess acid buildup, rendering the kidneys unable to keep up. Kidney stones are a form of acid waste that has not been properly removed because the body cannot eliminate the acid fast enough. These seemingly minor health concerns can be the first signs of more serious chronic health problems.

ACID OVERLOAD IN INFANTS

The negative effects of an acidic diet are not limited to adults. A 2001 German study demonstrated that preterm infants are at an especially high risk for acid overload because their kidneys are not capable of excreting the quantity of acid that is the result of eating common substandard infant formulas. The researchers linked this inability to properly filter and excrete excess acid with breathing irregularities, impaired growth, and a hormonal adaptation to bring the baby's body back to an acid–alkaline balance.[2] So it is important that infants are fed a highly alkaline diet of breast milk until they are old enough to begin eating mashed vegetables. And the food processing industry must be called to task to create better and more alkaline baby formulas. Nothing can replace breastfeeding for optimal infant nutrition, but breastfeeding is not always an option. Food corporations should not be allowed to compromise the health of babies. Parents need to pay more attention to what they put in their children's mouths, at least until children can make informed choices for themselves.

The Lungs and Other Detoxification Organs

The kidneys are key players in the fight against acidity, but they are not the body's only recourse. Our lungs remove carbon dioxide from our bodies as they maintain respiratory balance within our body systems. Increased oxygenation through deep breathing increases the oxygen in our blood and helps the body remove acid through the exhalation of carbon dioxide. That is why deep breathing techniques, meditation, yoga, qigong, and moderate aerobic exercise (the kind that does not cause a buildup of lactic acid in the muscles) are important.

Other detoxification organs, such as the liver, the intestines, and the skin, assist with acid–alkaline balance. The liver filters toxic compounds that may be acid-forming in the body. The intestines help expel acid by excreting it in our feces. And some acid is secreted through our skin when we perspire. When any of these mechanisms are dysfunctional, both the individual organs and the body as a whole are at risk of increased acid buildup.

The Lymphatic System

You might not know much about your lymphatic system, but it is critical to great health. The lymphatic system (or lymph system) is a complex network of fluid-filled nodes, glands, and tubes that bathe our cells and carry cellular waste to the bloodstream. In many ways, it is comparable to a street sweeper, sweeping up dirt and debris and carrying it out of our tissues. Your diet and lifestyle determine how quickly your lymphatic system eliminates acidic wastes.

The tonsils are part of the lymphatic system (they help prevent toxins from entering your body), as are the spleen and thymus. The lymphatic system handles toxins that enter your body from external sources, such as food or air pollution, but also deals with internally produced toxins (endotoxins), such as in inflammation, that are the result of normal metabolic processes. It carries acid waste products via lymph fluid, which enters your veins (and thus your bloodstream) near your heart. Once toxins have been swept up and dumped into the bloodstream, the kidneys and liver take over to filter them out of the blood.

A healthy lymphatic system also helps purify your blood. One of the ways it does this is through the largest mass of lymph tissue in the body, the spleen, an oval organ located to the left of the stomach, just under the lower part of your rib cage. The spleen fights bacteria, viruses, and other microbes that spew acid wastes as part of their metabolism.

There is three times more lymph fluid in the body than blood, yet it has no organ like the heart to pump it. That means it relies on deep breathing, movement, and massage to flow effectively. Stress plays a role in lymph flow, since we tend to breathe shallowly during stressful times. And if you drink inadequate amounts of water, as most people do, your lymphatic system will slow down; it requires fluid to function properly.

If your lymph system is inefficient, you may gain fatty deposits or cellulite, or experience aches and pains. A recent study found that 80 percent of overweight women have sluggish lymphatic systems, and that getting lymph fluid flowing smoothly is the key to easy weight loss and improved feelings of well-being.[3] In another study, Elisabeth Dancey, author of *The Cellulite Solution*, found that women with cellulite showed lymphatic system deficiencies.[4] (Cellulite, like other fatty deposits in the body, stores acidic wastes.) If you improve the cleansing ability of the lymph system, it will be able to sweep away the toxins that lead to cellulite. Many people who believe they are holding excess fat may actually be bloated due to a sluggish lymphatic system.

Neutralizing Acid

In addition to expelling acid, our bodies try to neutralize it by dumping naturally occurring substances such as calcium, potassium, bicarbonate, glutamine, and magnesium from our bones and muscles into our bloodstream.

The Bones

Let's take a look at one of the primary ways in which your body works to balance pH. Let's say that you, like most people in North America, eat an acid-forming diet. Perhaps your breakfast usually consists of a packaged cereal, milk, and coffee; you might take a mid-morning coffee break and eat a doughnut or croissant; your lunch might be a ham sandwich on whole wheat bread, with mayonnaise and mustard, accompanied by another coffee or cola; for dinner, you might eat a cheeseburger on a white bun, french fries, a cola, and a piece of cake. At some point in the day, you might have a couple of glasses of water and maybe another soda or two. With the possible exception of the water (which, depending on the source, may have been either acidic or alkaline), everything you've eaten on this average day creates acidity in the body.

Your kidneys will excrete some of this excess acidity. But if there is more than they can handle, another mechanism kicks in to put the brakes on and try to keep the blood at 7.365. This process centers around the bones, which the body uses as a sort of bank account system to maintain acid–alkaline balance. Whenever your body becomes excessively acidic, it makes a withdrawal of calcium from the bones, the primary storehouse of this very alkaline mineral, to neutralize the acidity. In its wisdom, the body knows that acidity can be disastrous; it will do whatever it can to prevent acidic blood from wreaking havoc on the many organs and organ systems it is supposed to nourish, including the brain.

Calcium withdrawn from our bones to combat acidity is dumped into our urine along with the acid expelled by our kidneys. A 2001 study by Dr. David Bushinsky proved that chronic acidity causes an increase in calcium excretion through the urine; however, no change in intestinal calcium absorption was observed (we absorb most nutrients, including calcium, through the walls of our intestines).[5] Because bone contains most of the body's calcium, it is widely regarded as the source of the increased calcium excretion in urine. This net loss of calcium is rarely reversed on the Standard American Diet. Nor can it be resolved simply by popping calcium pills. Unless we address the cause of the calcium loss—acidity—it is a lost battle.

While most of the discussion about acidity and bone loss focuses on calcium, the same study revealed that bone is also a reservoir for sodium and potassium, and its surface has receptor sites that normally bind with sodium, potassium, and hydrogen. When the body becomes too acidic, hydrogen bumps sodium and potassium off the bone surface to buffer the systemic acidity, further depleting the bones of minerals that are essential for their health and strength.

Though we expel carbon dioxide with every exhalation, some remains in our bones, bound to calcium, sodium, and other minerals. While most of it is relatively inaccessible, about a third is readily available to help our blood balance acidity. Sudden, short-term changes toward acidity in our bodies decrease the total amount of carbon dioxide that our bones can use to bind important minerals.

Dumping calcium and other substances from the bones might be a relatively harmless mechanism if it is rarely used, but it is not a sustainable approach to blood pH balance over the long term. Yet because of poor dietary and life-style patterns, that is precisely what most people are forcing their bodies to do. Balance may be restored to the blood, but it comes at a high cost: weakened bones and a suppressed capacity for additional bone formation. So it is no surprise that the incidence of bone-demineralizing diseases such as osteoporosis are on the rise. (You'll learn more about this tragic disorder in the next chapter.)

THE CALCIUM CONNECTION

Calcium is arguably involved in more biological functions than any other mineral. From bone health to muscle movement to our beating heart, calcium is critical on the cellular level. Calcium is also one of the most misrepresented and misunderstood minerals. We have all seen the advertisements touting calcium in everything from dairy products to heartburn tablets, coral supplements, and multi-mineral tablets. It is difficult to know what to believe and what to buy.

Calcium from clean, natural sources, such as fresh vegetables, has proven health benefits. We will talk about dairy products later in the book. Calcium supplements unadulterated by processing practices that involve chemicals or fillers (such as lead, which is found in many brands of calcium supplements) may be beneficial as well. Their effectiveness has as much to do with the body's capacity to assimilate and use the calcium as it does with the quantity of the calcium. If a product claim sounds too good to be true, chances are it is.

Certain cultures consume many times more than the recommended daily allowance of calcium suggested by modern medical health experts. In some cases, these people live at high altitudes and their drinking water comes from glacier-fed sources rich in calcium and other trace minerals. This calcium-rich water is also used for crop irrigation, so the plants contain higher levels of calcium too. Others, such as the highly publicized Okinawan island people of Japan, attribute some aspects of their health and longevity to the calcium-rich coral reefs. The Okinawan people are among the longest-living and healthiest people on the planet.

There are a few important facts you need to know about calcium:

1. Those of us who eat the Standard American Diet have a calcium deficiency for two main reasons: we don't eat enough biologically available calcium (that is, calcium that our bodies can use effectively to benefit our health), and we eat too many acid-forming foods, forcing our bodies to use up stored calcium to offset the acidity.
2. We can increase our consumption of biologically available calcium by eating more vegetables and legumes.
3. Dairy products, while a source of calcium, are acid-forming; therefore, they increase our calcium requirements.
4. Calcium helps to create oxygen at the cellular level, which aids in the prevention of disease and the creation of a more alkaline body.

The Muscles

In addition to reducing bone mass and strength, acidity can cause a loss of muscle protein when glutamine is released from skeletal muscle to restore the body's pH. Glutamine is an amino acid found in high–protein foods, such as fish, red meat, beans, and dairy products (many of which are acid-forming, but we will discuss solutions for this later in the book). In addition to being a constituent of proteins, glutamine is crucial for nitrogen metabolism in the body. Glutamine reduces acidity by binding hydrogen ions (electrically charged cells) to form ammonium (which is alkaline) in a process called nitrogen fixation. So glutamine acts in much the same way as calcium to neutralize acid. And, much like calcium, glutamine released from the muscles is excreted along with the acid, resulting in muscle loss.

The body will also sometimes dump magnesium, another alkaline mineral, from the muscles to help restore balance to the blood. Magnesium is required for a healthy heart, blood vessels, bones, teeth, muscles, hormones, nerves, and moods. It also activates hundreds of enzymes, allowing them to perform their critical functions in your body.

LONG-TERM BALANCE

So, in effect, there is truth to the medical belief that the human body has innate pH-balancing mechanisms. The body is miraculous in its ability to juggle trillions of functions every single second. However, it is erroneous to believe that the body can go on endlessly balancing blood pH without significant health ramifications. Most people have insufficient calcium and magnesium to support ongoing mineral dumps from their bones and muscles. Experts estimate that 79 percent of North Americans are deficient in calcium and 67 percent are deficient in magnesium. And these studies are looking only at recommended dietary allowances; they do not take into account the fact that our highly acidic diets increase our requirements of these minerals.

There is no easy way to measure acid–alkaline homeostasis in human beings unless the condition is an acute or chronic metabolic or respiratory acidosis. These are severe, life-threatening conditions and are not the focus of this book. Our bodies' systems are constantly shifting and adjusting to maintain the balance required to function. Consequently, our acid–alkaline balance can be out of whack even when there is no measurable change in blood pH or evidence that the body is doing something to buffer the acid.

While studies have shown that a healthy human's body systems continually compensate to maintain balance, they have also shown that net acid excretion continues after an acid-laden diet becomes more alkaline. In other words, the negative impact of a highly acidic diet continues to affect the body for some time after the diet improves, even if measurements show no detectable change in blood pH or carbon dioxide in the body. That's one reason why it is important to look at the Ultimate pH Solution as a lifestyle change and not a short-term fad.

pH Solution

Collette Conquers Fatigue

Collette was always tired. No amount of sleep helped. She dragged herself out of bed every morning and barely felt capable of handling her work and personal responsibilities during the day, even with three cups of coffee by noon. Her medical doctors ran tests on the functioning of her glands, but they all came back normal. Finally, they found that her iron levels were low, diagnosed her as anemic, and gave her iron supplements. She took her supplements faithfully, but the fatigue persisted. So she came to see me.

Since we already knew the results of her medical tests, I began by assessing Collette's diet and lifestyle. I suspected that her glands, although testing normal, were weakened by her acidic diet and chronic worrying. Also, she was drinking large amounts of coffee, which displaces iron from the body, counteracting the supplements. She rated her stress level as nine out of ten—very high. At my request, she wrote down everything she had eaten for the previous three days. I felt that her fatigue was a sign of a deeper imbalance and suspected that her acidic food choices were finally catching up with her.

After reviewing her food diary, I could see that almost everything she ate was creating acidity in her body. After hitting the snooze button a few times every morning, Collette never had time for a good breakfast. Instead, she hit the Starbucks drive-through for a coffee and muffin. For lunch, she sampled the food court's "healthy" options—usually macaroni or potato salad smothered in a mayonnaise dressing, chili with tortilla chips, or a bagel with cream cheese. Dinner might consist of a Lean Cuisine lasagna with meat sauce or a take-out taco salad from her local Mexican restaurant.

Collette explained that she had no energy to make meals or shop for groceries. I understood. Lack of energy and lack of understanding about what constitutes healthy food can create a vicious cycle that causes acidity and more fatigue. I asked Collette to increase her alkaline food choices for the next month, and she agreed. In place of her morning coffee habit, she began drinking green tea sweetened with stevia and then added a large glass of water with lemon juice after a few days. She took her iron supplements at least one hour prior to drinking the tea to ensure absorption. On Sunday nights, she threw all the ingredients for Slow Cooker Black Bean Chili (page 164) into her slow cooker so it was ready to take to work on Monday morning. It could also be reheated for an easy weeknight dinner. She kept jars of Herb Dressing and Blueberry Dressing (page 160) in the fridge along with a large package of organic salad greens for quick light lunches. Once she had more time and energy, she explored more of the recipes I gave her.

After a month, Collette returned to my office with a skip in her step. She admitted that the first week had been difficult. She'd had to adjust to life without coffee, and she wasn't used to making home-cooked meals. But her newfound energy and improved sleep more than made up for the energy it took to cook and change her dietary habits. She told a friend about her new lifestyle, and they decided to make large batches of different recipes and share them. This made food preparation easier for both of them and brought them closer. Collette also started going to a yoga studio, which helped to alleviate her chronic worry and introduced her to some like-minded friends.

CHAPTER 3

The Acid–Disease Connection

"Faced with the choice between changing one's mind and proving there is no need to do so, almost everyone gets busy on the proof."

—JOHN KENNETH GALBRAITH

Frank, a 47-year-old chief financial officer at a high-tech company, came to me to see if I could help him with his chronic headaches. He typically suffered four every week, and they were interfering with his work. After reviewing his diet and lifestyle, I knew that his stressful job played a role, but my instincts told me that his cola addiction played an even greater one. When I suggested that he eliminate Coca-Cola from his diet, I could see his tension grow. "Eliminate?" he asked in disbelief. He knew cola was unhealthy, but he enjoyed it so much that he couldn't imagine never having it again.

After further discussion, we compromised. Frank agreed to drink lemon water, eat more vegetables, and drink green drinks if he could have cola as a treat once a week. It gave him something to look forward to on the weekends, and helped keep him motivated the rest of the time. On the day that he had his cola, he made sure to drink extra lemon water and green drinks throughout the day to restore his pH as quickly as possible. He also signed up at a gym to work off some of the stress associated with his job. Soon, Frank was experiencing a headache only once every two to three weeks, and he admitted that he had started to enjoy the food, the green drinks, and even the vegetables! He found the diet completely manageable—as long as he knew he could enjoy a weekend cola.

Like Frank, you may be needlessly suffering from headaches or some other ailment linked to an unbalanced pH. Let's take a look at some of the other health issues related to excess acid in our bodies.

DISEASES AND SYMPTOMS

The typical nutrient-poor and highly acidic diet can throw off the delicate balance in our bodies, resulting in unhealthy cells. Unhealthy cells can lead to the growth of damaging pathogens, which, through their very survival, release more acid wastes, which damage even more cells. The body attempts to adapt to this acidic environment, but as it maintains this unhealthy cycle it begins to experience negative symptoms. These symptoms are then diagnosed as diseases, though they are really signs of an underlying pH imbalance. Even cancer tumors are symptoms of the unhealthy, oxygen-deprived, acidic environment underlying them. More than that, even the germs that are considered to be the cause of various illnesses are symptoms of the unhealthy, acidic environment in which they thrive.

A growing number of groundbreaking studies, published in popular, recognized scientific journals, link a wide range of health disorders to an acidic state in the body. Some of the conditions most commonly associated with excess acid formation include arthritis, kidney disease, osteoporosis, weight gain, and chronic infections such as sinusitis and bronchitis. Most shocking, perhaps, is that cancer is increasingly being added to this list.

The diseases, disorders, and conditions listed in the following box have more in common than a link to acidity. They are also health problems that modern medicine has not been particularly effective at curing. The Western medical approach to disease is often called a "Band-Aid approach" because it addresses only symptoms rather than the root causes of a condition. This criticism is valid, but the Band-Aid image does not truly reflect the potential danger. When it comes to many serious health concerns, the Western approach might be more accurately described as an attempt to cork a volcano: it might stop the flow of lava for the moment, but the problem still exists and will likely lead to a more explosive and deadly incident in the future. Similarly, masking symptoms with drugs may alleviate certain conditions temporarily, but if the underlying problem is never addressed, it will more often than not rear its ugly head in the form of a more serious disease at a future date.

Now that we know these diseases, disorders, and conditions have been linked with acidity, and that drugs are not actually curing them, let's examine the role acidity plays in a handful of the more common health problems on the list.

DISEASES AND CONDITIONS LINKED TO ACIDITY

Here's an expanded list of the disorders that researchers are linking to acidity. This list is extensive, but probably not exhaustive.

- Allergies
- Alzheimer's disease
- Amyotrophic lateral sclerosis (also known as Lou Gehrig's disease)
- Arteriosclerosis
- Arthritis
- Bone fractures
- Bronchitis
- Cancer
- Candidiasis
- Cardiovascular disease
- Chronic fatigue syndrome
- Chronic infections
- Dementia
- Depression
- Diabetes
- Fibromyalgia
- Heart attacks
- High blood pressure
- High cholesterol
- Hormonal imbalances
- Immune deficiencies
- Insulin insensitivity
- Kidney disease
- Multiple sclerosis
- Muscular dystrophy
- Obesity
- Osteoarthritis
- Osteoporosis
- Parkinson's disease
- Premature aging
- Premature hair graying
- Prostate problems
- Senility
- Sinusitis
- Stroke
- Tooth decay and loss of teeth
- Weight problems

Allergies

Allergies are commonplace in our industrialized society, but that does not make them normal. I rarely encounter a client who doesn't exhibit allergy symptoms or sensitivity to at least one thing. Allergy symptoms such as a stuffy nose, sneezing, and itchy, red eyes used to be associated only with common allergens found in nature, such as goldenrod, ragweed, pollen, and pets. These days, however, more and more people are experiencing a broad range of allergy-like symptoms triggered by chemicals, food, and pollutants.

An overly acidic environment creates a breeding ground for toxins. Acidity goes hand in hand with oxygen deprivation, and an oxygen-deprived environment allows harmful microorganisms such as bacteria, viruses, and fungi to flourish. While there are some beneficial microorganisms, the majority are toxic, as are their metabolic wastes. They continually stress the immune system and can eventually exhaust it. In this state, the body becomes ultra-sensitive to chemicals, foods, pollen, and other foreign substances, and it reacts by making the eyes water, the nose run, and the tissues swell, or worse. The body's efforts to eliminate acidic waste products are at best uncomfortable and at worst life-threatening.

Allergic reactions and other immune responses also generate huge amounts of acidic by-products, which can create a dangerous cycle for the allergy sufferer—a cycle that can be stopped by restoring the blood to a slightly alkaline state.

Alzheimer's and Other Age-Related Diseases

The *European Journal of Nutrition* links aging and age-related disorders to acid–alkaline imbalances.[1] In my book *The Brain Wash*, I discuss the dangers of exposure to heavy metals and pesticides, as well as the damage caused by alcohol consumption. These substances contribute to excess acidity in the body as our systems try to metabolize, neutralize, or eliminate them. Once they are in our bodies, it can be difficult to get rid of them. They promote inflammation and increase the formation of free radicals (charged molecules that attack healthy tissues). Both inflammation and free radicals are associated with brain diseases such as Alzheimer's.

Elevated levels of the hormone homocysteine, a by-product of protein digestion and metabolism, have been linked to age-related diseases such as heart disease and Alzheimer's. Research shows that by reducing our consumption of acidic protein foods, such as meat, we may be able to reduce and control our homocysteine levels. Studies have also shown that the B vitamins B_6, B_{12}, niacin, and folate can help lower levels of homocysteine in the blood.[2]

A study published in the journal *Neurological Research* found that blood cells in the brain were heavily damaged by a slightly acidic state (6.6 pH). The researchers believe that acidity may play an important role in the development of dementia and Alzheimer's disease.[3]

Arthritis

The 143 joints in the human body require a slightly alkaline environment to stay healthy and strong. Without that environment, they begin to deteriorate and become vulnerable to various injuries and illnesses, including arthritis. At least one in three adults in the United States currently suffers from chronic joint symptoms or arthritis, and the Public Health Agency of Canada estimates that 85 percent of Canadians will be affected by osteoarthritis by age 70.

There are numerous forms of arthritis, including fibromyalgia, gout, lupus, and scleroderma. The two most common types are osteoarthritis and rheumatoid arthritis. Osteoarthritis is a joint disease, but rheumatoid arthritis damages the connective tissue and is considered an autoimmune disease, meaning that the body's immune system mistakenly attacks healthy tissue, not just pathogens such as viruses or bacteria.

A growing body of research illustrates the link between acidic diets and arthritis. The health of your joints is based on many factors, one of which is a stable blood pH. If blood pH becomes excessively acidic, it can cause inflammation, and inflammation can damage joints. In some studies, researchers were even able to *produce* inflammation comparable to arthritis in the joints of animals simply by switching their water to milk.[4] Milk does a body good? Certainly not for people with acid buildup in their blood and joints. As you learned in chapter 1, milk creates acidity in the body. Many of the factors that are known to increase acidity also cause systemic inflammation, including joint inflammation. Acidity and inflammation go hand in hand.

Our joints contain cartilage, a gelatinous tissue that, like all body tissues, is made up of cells. And, like most cells, cartilage cells require a slightly alkaline environment to function properly. This environment is balanced by a combination of salts and water, which pulls acid out of the cartilage cells and washes it away. High acidity can dehydrate cartilage, killing cells and undermining the joint's ability to create new tissue. This leads to greater friction around the joint and the pain and inflammation associated with osteoarthritis.

Studies have demonstrated that feeding a high-fat diet to animals that are susceptible to autoimmune diseases increased the severity of rheumatoid arthritis.[5] Conversely, studies have shown that a vegetarian, gluten-free diet improved symptoms of rheumatoid arthritis.[6] Most high-fat diets are largely acidic, while vegetarian diets tend to have a higher ratio of alkaline foods.

Many of my patients have gotten relief from arthritis simply by eliminating toxins from their lifestyle and eating a more alkaline diet like the one outlined later in this book. In addition, people who take Aspirin for arthritis pain may want to explore other options: Aspirin and other pain-relief drugs that contain salicylates are known to increase acidity in the body. (Remember that Aspirin's chemical name is acetylsalicylic *acid*.)

Bone Fractures

We often think of bones as non-living, concrete-like substances that have little to do other than support us. But bones are alive—as much as any other tissue in the body. And they are integral to our overall health. Blood cells are manufactured in bone marrow, which makes bones just as important to body function as they are to body structure: our heart, lungs, kidneys, muscles, and everything else need a constant supply of healthy blood. Bones also act as holding places for essential chemical elements. Excess nutrients are either excreted in the urine or deposited on the bones. When the body has a shortage of a particular nutrient, it can draw upon the bones to replenish its stores, sending the nutrient where it is needed most. The minerals calcium, phosphorus, and magnesium, for example, are stored in the bones in large quantities. On average, our bones contain about 1.4 kilograms of calcium, 680 milligrams of phosphorus, and 25 milligrams of magnesium. Almost 99 percent of the body's calcium is found in the bones.[7]

We take the many functions of our bones for granted until we fracture one and feel the excruciating pain as our body alerts us to the injury. When a bone fractures, we become intimately aware of the vital role our bones play in maintaining our body's balance, our posture, and our overall health.

Research in a number of medical publications, such as the *European Journal of Nutrition*, links bone disorders such as fractures to acid–base imbalances.[8] In his book *Beautiful Bones Without Hormones*, Dr. Leon Root states, "Even a small drop in the body's pH can cause a dramatic increase in bone loss."[9] Remember that a drop in pH means an increase in acidity.

Cancer

Perhaps more than other disease, cancer is a reflection of our modern environmental and lifestyle choices. The World Health Organization (WHO) publishes the *World Cancer Report*, which documents cancer trends, the frequency of cancer in different countries, and mortality rates. Their research suggests that approximately 4 percent of cancers are inherited or genetic; the rest are preventable and are linked to lifestyle, diet, and the environment.

All living organisms, humans included, are electrical beings. Every healthy cell in the human body carries a measurable electromagnetic negative charge. Cells in an acidic, oxygen-deprived environment have an electromagnetic positive charge. Because the laws of electromagnetism demand that opposites attract, unhealthy cells and their acid attract and bind to healthy cells. This increases the likelihood that healthy cells will be damaged by the acidic environment or by the cell fermentation process that occurs when inadequate oxygen is available for healthy cell function. As the mass of unhealthy tissue grows, the body often creates a defense mechanism to surround and isolate the tissue in an effort to prevent its spread. In cancer, this is referred to as a tumor.[10]

Cancer cells can form from normal cells when DNA and/or RNA is modified or mutated, either spontaneously or as a result of any number of external factors, including radiation, chemicals and toxins, pathogens (bacteria, viruses, fungi, and parasites), and the water and food we ingest. If the immune system is not functioning properly or is overburdened, cancer cells can proliferate and effectively overpower its capacity to destroy them.

Many holistically-minded health experts consider cancer an effect of deep imbalances in the body, not a disease. These imbalances are caused by metabolic acids that build up in the blood and are released into cells, tissues, and organs.

Whatever your view on cancer, an abundance of research links the Standard American Diet and its inherent acidity to numerous forms of cancer. Food and water provide fuel for our bodies and feed us on the cellular level. If the fuel is excessively acidic, it builds an unhealthy cell environment, opening the door for mutations. Acidity reduces oxygen, and cancer thrives in an oxygen-poor, acid-rich environment. Cancer cells can obtain energy through fermentation, a conversion process that does not require oxygen. While normal cells can no longer divide and survive in this type of environment, cancer cells flourish on the few available nutrients.

In 1931, the German physiologist and medical doctor Otto Warburg was awarded the Nobel Prize for his research on the nature and action of respiratory enzymes. He focused on the metabolism of tumors and cells and was particularly interested in cancer cells. Warburg's hypothesis, published in *The Prime Cause and Prevention of Cancer*, suggested that anaerobiosis—a process of energy production in a cell with no oxygen present—was a primary cause of cancerous cells.

Today, many health professionals claim that Otto Warburg found the cure for cancer. They believe that the medical profession simply ignores his findings to sustain the cancer research industry. This is a bit of a stretch, in my opinion, but Warburg's work is critical to our understanding of cancer growth, cell oxygenation, and the role pH plays in creating a healthy cellular environment that is resistant to cancer and other diseases.

Researchers have recently found evidence that links impaired mitochondrial function to the spread of cancer cells.[11] Found in cells, mitochondria convert food molecules into energy. Without adequate energy, our cells can find it hard to stave off cancer. When this evidence is combined with Warburg's hypothesis regarding cell respiration, today's scientists have a greater understanding of how cancer cells grow, divide, and expand.

Still, most cancer research is directed at drug development and invasive treatments rather than at the role of food and nutrition in cancer prevention. Ignoring food, nutrition, and lifestyle options that would prevent many cancers helps sustain the cancer industry. If a mere 10 percent of the money used for researching drugs as a possible treatment for cancer was invested in educating people in healthy eating and lifestyle choices, we would see measurable progress in the seemingly hopeless fight against cancer and many other diseases. Many cancers would be prevented before they could even form. Even the conservative estimates by the Centers for Disease Control and Prevention link 30 percent of cancers to diet.

So why is Warburg's hypothesis regarding cell respiration, cancer, and anaerobiosis important to the discussion of acidity? Alkaline solutions generally absorb oxygen, while acidic solutions expel oxygen. Our bodies are mildly alkaline by nature, as are our bodily fluids, with the exception of digestive juices and urine. Blood, for example, must remain in a very narrow alkaline range, around pH 7.4, to retain its oxygen. When the body becomes acidic thanks to a diet lacking sufficient minerals and nutrients, its natural mechanisms start to search out minerals and nutrients from the organs to maintain pH at 7.4. The cells of these organs become acidic, and their capacity to take up oxygen—cell respiration—is compromised. In the absence of adequate oxygen, cells seek energy by converting glucose through fermentation, which produces more acid and further lowers the pH of the cells. This creates an environment in which cancer cells can grow and multiply even as the body tries to correct the pH imbalance.

Researchers at the Centre for Mathematical Biology at the University of Oxford found that both acidity and a lack of oxygen are factors in the evolution of non-malignant tumors to invasive cancers.[12] Researchers at the Department of Radiotherapy/Oncology at Democritus University of Thrace Medical School in Greece found very low pH levels (which you'll recall means acid) in the veins of cancerous tumors of the gastrointestinal tract, suggesting that these tumors are intensely acidic.[13] Still other research shows that the cells of most solid tumors are surrounded by acid.[14]

While reducing the acid in our bodies is no guarantee that we'll never experience cancer, by doing so we may be cutting off cancer cells from the very means to their survival. Remember that changing the body's pH is not a cure-all for disease; instead, it allows the body to heal itself by enabling it to function optimally so that toxins, including cancer cells, can be eliminated before they amass. Cancer cells exist even in a healthy body. But healthy bodies are able to kill and remove cancer and other diseased cells before they can build up to form tumors. When you follow the holistic Kick Acid approach to health, your body returns to optimal functionality, minimizing the likelihood of cancer, and of disease in general.

Candidiasis

There are numerous forms of candida, but when discussing the fungal overgrowth candidiasis, we are usually referring to *Candida albicans*. While it is a fungus, it is more commonly called a yeast. It occurs naturally in our gastrointestinal tract and plays an important role in our health: we need candida in the right amount to be healthy. However, the typical North American diet causes candida to proliferate out of control, resulting in overgrowth that can cause yeast infections, thrush (candida growing in the throat), fatigue, headaches, mood swings, irritability, cravings, bloating, indigestion, allergic reactions, and countless other symptoms. As unbelievable as it sounds, extreme cases of candidiasis have even resulted in death.

Because it is a living thing—a single-cell plant, in fact—candida produces and releases waste, and its waste is toxic and acidic. Over 80 different toxins that break down tissue in the body have been linked to candida overgrowth. For example, candida can weaken the mucous membrane of the gut, causing leakage. Undigested proteins and other foreign bodies can then be absorbed into the bloodstream, leading to allergic reactions and food or chemical sensitivities. In my experience, candidiasis is also a common underlying factor in autoimmune disorders such as rheumatoid arthritis and fibromyalgia.

Thanks to the typical diet, full of acid-forming meat and dairy products and loaded with sugars, candidiasis and other overgrowths of yeasts and fungus are an epidemic. It would be unusual to find a person eating this diet who did not have a fungal overgrowth. The Standard American Diet feeds and fuels these opportunistic organisms even more than it feeds and fuels the health-sustaining cells in our bodies. Candida thrives in an acidic environment, and it creates more acidity just by being alive.

The symptoms of candidiasis and fungal overgrowth are extensive: fatigue, digestive problems and bloating, headaches, pain, inflammation, depression, hyperactivity, respiratory problems, susceptibility to colds and flu, infections, growth of cysts and tumors—the list is seemingly endless. Many experienced practitioners in the natural health field suggest that most disease and degeneration can be traced to an overgrowth of bacteria, yeast, fungus, mold, or other microforms and the acidic wastes they excrete in the body. While it is true that many people with poor health are suffering from an overgrowth of candida or another type of microbe, I believe that the overgrowth is merely a side effect of an acidic body. Eliminate the acidity, and you cut off these harmful microbes from their food source, ultimately starving them to death.

Chronic Fatigue Syndrome

In 2006, the Centers for Disease Control and Prevention (CDC), a recognized authority on disease, launched a highly public media and education campaign to announce that chronic fatigue syndrome (CFS), or myalgic encephalomyelitis, is a serious, scientifically validated disease. It is characterized by severe, disabling fatigue lasting for more than six months, associated with physical and mental disturbances such as headaches, joint pain, muscle pain, memory impairment, sore throat, and tender lymph nodes. It is a debilitating and frequently disabling disease, and the medical community, as well as the public, must follow the CDC's lead by acknowledging chronic fatigue syndrome as they would any other disease. For too long, many doctors, employers, and even friends and family have belittled the real and disabling symptoms suffered by individuals afflicted with CFS. Because there are so many causative factors yet few definitive medical tests for this disease, many people incorrectly assumed that the disease was a product of the sufferer's imagination. But research has increasingly demonstrated severe biochemical and neurological abnormalities in sufferers with CFS.

Now that the CDC has publicly legitimized CFS and helped validate the suffering of so many people, it will be interesting to see if additional research funds and efforts are directed toward this disease. To date, CFS has been linked to viral infections, immune system damage, nutritional deficiencies, impaired detoxification systems, pathogens, fungal and bacterial overgrowth in the intestines, chemical sensitivities, chronic high stress levels, pharmaceutical drugs and vaccines, impaired neurological function, and poor adrenal function.

Perhaps even more than cancer, CFS is a reflection of the impact our modern toxic environment has on the human body. In chapter 1, we learned how processed foods, dairy products, meat, refined sugars, and food additives such as aspartame can increase the acidity in our bodies. People with CFS are very susceptible to these substances, and their vulnerability manifests as food allergies, environmental sensitivities, and increased permeability of the blood–brain barrier, a protective mechanism designed to keep harmful substances from damaging the brain. But what came first? Could the exposure to and consumption of these toxic and acidic substances tax a person's body enough to chronically suppress detoxification organs and ultimately the immune system, rendering it incapable of dealing with toxicity and acidity? For everyone, there is a point after which the body can no longer handle the volume of toxins to which it has been exposed—called the toxic load, or body burden. This might explain how someone can be fine one day and then wake up the next to face debilitating symptoms: his or her body can no longer deal with the toxic load.

Researchers at the Department of Infectious Diseases at G. d'Annunzio University in Chieti Scalo, Italy, studied the possible factors that trigger the onset of CFS. Their findings substantiate what many sufferers of CFS already know: an exposure to chemical and/or food toxins is frequently a precipitating factor for the disease.[15]

Acidity allows the viruses associated with this disease to flourish, particularly the Epstein–Barr virus. It overloads the detoxification mechanisms and shuts down production of critical enzymes, thereby preventing proper detoxification of toxins linked to the disease. It can interfere with the uptake of nutrients, leading to the deficiencies that are common in CFS. Furthermore, chronic acidity can reduce the functionality of critical glands, such as the adrenal glands, a frequent problem for sufferers of CFS.

Depression

We all get down at some point in our lives, but the World Health Organization estimates that 10 percent of the population has symptoms that are significant enough to require medical attention. In this type of depression, physical and psychological symptoms significantly reduce a person's functionality for a prolonged period of time. The depressed person also exhibits sadness that seems disproportionate to the apparent cause.

Many of the symptoms of depression are similar to those of an acidic body or one in which pathogenic overgrowth has taken hold. Acid-forming substances such as alcohol, recreational drugs, heavy metals and other chemicals, food additives and colors, processed foods, trans fats, sugars, and pharmaceutical drugs have been implicated in depression.

Hormonal imbalances are often linked with depression, and rapid blood sugar fluctuations are often linked with hormonal imbalances. When we consume acidic, high-sugar products and alcohol, we can throw our blood sugar out of whack, triggering a series of events that ultimately disrupts our hormone levels.

I worked with a patient who could not figure out why she occasionally felt suicidal. She had never been diagnosed with clinical depression or any other form of mental illness, and these rare thoughts were out of sync with her normally cheerful disposition. She was reluctant to take medication or undergo psychiatric counseling because she didn't feel depressed and didn't subscribe to this approach. She described her suicidal thoughts as arising "out of nowhere," which I believed because, other than this one serious concern, she seemed quite happy.

As we tried to analyze her situation, she mentioned that her suicidal thoughts always followed consumption of fudge or other sweets. Fudge is loaded with sugar, which causes rapid blood sugar spikes that come crashing down soon afterward. Her mood followed suit. Once she eliminated blood sugar–altering sweets and began eating a more alkaline diet, she lost her cravings for sweets. More importantly, her moods balanced, she no longer had suicidal thoughts, and her vibrant personality was able to shine. Depression no longer had a hold on her.

While there is little research on the connection between acidity and depression, I have personally witnessed dramatic improvements in many previously depressed individuals who switched their diet to a more alkaline one. I anticipate that future studies on the topic will demonstrate the connection. In the meantime, you can benefit, as many others have, from the mood-balancing effects of a more alkaline diet.

Diabetes

More than 18 million people in the United States suffer from diabetes. In Canada, the number is between 2 and 3 million, and growing rapidly. A Canadian study published in *Lancet* in 2007 suggested that the disease is outpacing growth expectations, with no signs of slowing down. Lorraine Lipscombe of the Institute for Clinical Evaluative Sciences in Toronto found that the percentage of people with diabetes in Ontario—Canada's most populous province—has jumped noticeably. It now affects 8.8 percent of the population, or about one in every 11 adults; in 1995, it affected just 5.2 percent, or one in every 19 people. The study suggests that rising obesity levels across North America are contributing to the onset of the disease.[16]

There are two types of diabetes. In Type 1 diabetes, the pancreas produces no insulin on its own, or almost none, and the individual is dependent on insulin injections for life. In Type 2 diabetes, which is usually the result of poor eating habits, the pancreas does not produce enough insulin, and the body's ability to use that insulin is impaired. In either case, it is critical for people with diabetes to maintain blood glucose levels within a certain range and avoid the massive blood sugar fluctuations caused by eating sweets.

In addition to insulin (a hormone that moves blood sugar into cells for energy production, helping to regulate blood glucose levels), the pancreas produces the most alkaline fluid in the body, a fluid loaded with digestive enzymes. In an acidic environment, the growth of yeasts, molds, and fungi can compromise the pancreas's function and damage the body's ability to metabolize sugar.

According to the Canadian Diabetes Association, four out of five people with diabetes die of heart disease. Other complications of diabetes include kidney and nerve damage, blindness, and sexual dysfunction. A study conducted by the University of Texas Southwestern Medical Center in Dallas found that people with Type 2 diabetes have highly acidic urine and are at greater risk of developing uric acid kidney stones.[17]

Over the course of a six-month controlled study, biochemist Robert O. Young studied the effects of specific alkaline foods, aerobic exercise, and nutritional supplements on people with Type 1 or Type 2 diabetes. His results were astonishing. In every case, he found that the people who completed the study were able to decrease or discontinue their medications, including cutting their insulin intake by over 50 percent or eliminating it altogether. The individuals participating in his study lost weight (an average of 32 pounds after the first 12 weeks), lowered their blood pressure, and reduced their total cholesterol.[18] Working in conjunction with the University of Miami, Dr. Young is now conducting similar research on a much larger group of people with diabetes.

Infection

Acidity is the favored environment of microorganisms of all kinds, including bacteria, viruses, yeasts, fungi, and molds. These critters require an acidic environment to live, grow, thrive, and multiply. The 19th-century French physiologist Claude Bernard aptly stated, "Illnesses hover constantly above us, their seed blown by the winds, but they do not set in the terrain unless the terrain is ready to receive them."[19] In other words, viruses, bacteria, and other germs are not nearly as dangerous when the body is in balance, but they begin to take hold when we become acidic. This thesis is supported by none other than Louis Pasteur, the chemist who brought the world the pasteurization process. Pasteur felt that the best way to fight germs was to inhibit their formation in a substance such as milk (hence the term "pasteurization"). It is believed, however, that later in his life Pasteur admitted, "The germ is nothing; the terrain is everything." Pasteur recognized that the body has greater success against germs when it is equipped to fight them. And the best way to equip the body is to restore its natural, slightly alkaline state.

An excessively acidic environment allows the microbes that give us influenza (flu), colds, sinusitis, bronchitis, and other viral and bacterial infections to proliferate. Many people find themselves coming down with one of these illnesses after the holiday season and assume that they've "caught" something that was "going around." Don't blame the guests you invited for dinner, blame the acidic foods you ate: turkey, stuffing, mashed potatoes, bread, butter, gravy, cranberry sauce, pie, and ice cream = acid, acid, and more acid.

Microbes love the low oxygen levels that come with acidity in the body. To make matters worse, these creatures secrete poisonous acid by-products that increase acidity—and the likelihood that they will continue to propagate at your health's expense. And their nefarious behavior doesn't stop there: to produce these acids, the microbes digest and ferment the very energy sources our body needs for cellular functions. So not only do they emit poisons that damage our health but they rob us of necessary energy at the same time.

Microbes can rapidly change their form and function. Bacteria can become yeasts, yeasts can change into fungi, and fungi can turn into molds. This ability to evolve is called pleomorphism, a long word that basically just means "many forms." Biochemist Robert O. Young has witnessed and recorded the mutation of bacteria into yeasts, then into fungi and molds, and ultimately back into bacteria. His research has led to his theory that our blood cells can do the same thing: de-evolve and then re-evolve to become cells the body requires, such as bone cells, brain cells, skin cells, heart cells, or muscle cells. Dr. Young has also seen human blood cells in acidic conditions turn into microbes such as bacteria.[20] While this sounds like something out of a science fiction movie, it is indicative of just how damaging blood acidity can be.

Kidney Disease

Studies published in the *American Journal of Kidney Disease* and *Kidney International*, among others, link acidity to kidney disease.[21] As we learned in chapter 2, the kidneys are important detoxification organs. They convert waste products and excess water to urine, producing 1½ to 2½ quarts of urine each day. They help the body balance chemicals and minerals, and they produce hormones that help regulate blood pressure and red blood cell production. These mighty little organs also help monitor the acidity of our blood.

An acidic system introduces unusually high levels of waste into the kidneys for filtration. If the kidneys cannot keep up, the waste accumulates and can form kidney stones (which are composed primarily of salts made up of uric acid and phosphoric acid) or get into the bloodstream and lead to inflammation elsewhere in the body. Damaged kidneys cannot maintain normal acidity levels and chemical balance in the body. This vicious cycle leads to disease and, if left unchecked, can result in kidney failure.

Many people wrongly assume that kidney stones are caused by excess calcium in the body. The real culprit may be excessive levels of phosphoric acid, the primary ingredient in cola and other sodas. The body uses calcium it leaches from the bones to convert phosphoric acid into a more stable form called phosphate. Phosphates can form into calcified kidney stones.[22] Researchers have found that patients who drink more alkaline mineral water containing bicarbonate see a reduction in uric acid kidney stones.[23]

Kidney and urinary tract diseases affect over 20 million Americans and result in an estimated 100,000 deaths each year. It is very difficult to detect kidney problems at an early stage because the symptoms can seem vague: fatigue, frequent urination, and even depression—all of which can be ascribed to numerous other causes. If you suspect kidney problems, it's best to consult your physician and follow the Ultimate pH Solution.

Osteoporosis

Acidity plays a significant role in the progression of osteoporosis, a disease that currently affects more than 25 million Americans, 80 percent of whom are women. Bone fractures are common in people suffering from osteoporosis, and more than 20,000 people die every year as a result of hip fractures.[24] By 2020, one in two Americans older than 50 will be at risk for fractures from osteoporosis or low bone mass, according to the U.S. Surgeon General.[25]

The bones are your body's calcium bank account. You know what would happen if you regularly withdrew money from your bank account and rarely made deposits: you'd eventually run out of cash. The same is true of your bones. Your body can't keep withdrawing calcium from the bones to neutralize acidity in your blood without serious repercussions. When excess consumption of acid-forming foods causes higher mineral loss from the bones than can be reabsorbed through mineral consumption, a mineral deficit occurs. If this net loss continues over a long period of time, the disturbing result can be osteoporosis: porous bones.

You may be thinking, "I can just eat more dairy products. After all, they build strong bones." That's what conventional medical thought and the various dairy bureaus that market and profit from dairy products would have you believe, but it couldn't be further from the truth. Dairy products are high in concentrated proteins that cause acidity in the body. Scientists link a high-protein diet from meat and dairy products to bone demineralization. Consuming dairy products can cause the body to lose more calcium from the bones than it can take in.

Harvey Diamond, nutrition expert and author of *Fit for Life*, says, "In the same way that we have been conditioned to think of meat whenever the word 'protein' is mentioned, we have also been taught to believe that dairy products are the finest source of calcium, and the best means by which to prevent osteoporosis. That is precisely what the dairy industry, which makes billions of dollars selling dairy products, wants you to believe, and once again, is patently untrue." He adds, "The countries of the world that consume the greatest amount of dairy products have the highest incidence of osteoporosis! The countries that consume the lowest amount of dairy products have the lowest incidence of osteoporosis."[26]

According to Walter C. Willett, chairman of the Department of Nutrition at the Harvard School of Public Health, "There's no solid evidence that merely increasing the amount of milk in your diet will protect you from breaking a hip or wrist or crushing a backbone in later years."[27] Willett's team at Harvard has been conducting research on the topic for the past 25 years. Willet is one of the principal investigators in two key studies: the Nurses' Health Study, which has looked at the diet and health of tens of thousands of nurses since 1976, and the Health Professionals Follow-Up Study, an all-male study under way since 1986. When Willett and his colleagues investigated the milk-drinking habits of 72,000 women in the Nurses' Health Study, they found that milk consumption was *not* associated with a lower risk of hip fracture, a measure of bone strength.[28] Likewise, the Health Professionals Follow-Up Study failed to find a relationship between calcium intake from dairy products and bone fractures in more than 43,000 men.[29]

T. Colin Campbell, professor emeritus of nutritional biochemistry at Cornell University, agrees that dairy products don't build bones. In an article for the *Los Angeles Times*, he said, "I like dairy. I grew up on a farm. But one has to look at the facts. . . . Dairy has been considered a health food, and that's an unfortunate myth."[30] Campbell and his colleagues at Cornell conducted a series of studies that are collectively known as the China Study. He has published the results in book form under the same name. He found that Asians, who consume far less dietary calcium than Americans, have one-fifth the bone fracture rate. Campbell says, "Those countries that use the most cow's milk and its products also have the highest fracture rates and the worst bone health."[31] In Asian countries, he notes, people get all the calcium their bodies need from plant sources, such as leafy green vegetables. He believes that Americans have weak bones because they drink excessive amounts of milk, and that animal protein, including that found in milk, makes blood and tissues more acidic. To neutralize this acid, the body leaches calcium from the bones.

The Cornell and Harvard studies are relatively recent, but research from as far back as the 1920s has shown that protein from meat and dairy products causes a net loss of calcium. The multi-billion-dollar dairy industry has kept this finding under wraps, instead indoctrinating us with "Milk does a body good" campaigns featuring celebrities sporting the finest milk moustaches. Don't be fooled. The dairy industry is powerful, and huge sums of money are at stake. The dairy industry in Idaho alone is worth approximately $1.5 billion. And dairy bureaus and associations spend hundreds of millions of dollars on marketing. With that kind of money going toward advertising the so-called health benefits of cow's milk, it's no surprise that people believe it is essential to bone health. Got milk? If so, you might want to reconsider your choice.

Medical researchers are not limiting their studies to dairy products alone. A study published in the *American Journal of Clinical Nutrition* links high meat consumption to an increased rate of bone density loss and an increased incidence of fractures.[32] Another study in the same journal found that cola consumption contributes to low bone-mineral density.[33] Similarly, research published in *Osteoporosis International* links increased cola consumption with adverse bone effects and a possible increase in the risk of osteoporosis, even in the short term.[34]

Acid-forming foods are not the only culprits in bone-mineral depletion. Depression and stress also contribute to osteoporosis. A recent *ABC News* report stated, "Growing evidence suggests that depression, one of the most common diseases of the brain, is so powerful it can actually erode bones in the body."[35] Stress hormones, like those secreted in depressed individuals or people with chronically stressful lives, are acid-forming. Excess amounts of these hormones deplete bone minerals, resulting in fragile bones. The body's primary stress hormone, cortisol, is extremely acidic and has an acidifying effect on the body's pH balance.[36] Stress hormones increase inflammatory signals called eicosanoids, which disrupt bone-building signals and communication.

Research published in the *American Journal of Physiology—Renal Physiology* found that stress, and the resulting elevated cortisol levels, slowed bone building and contributed dramatically to the breakdown of bones.[37]

To keep your bones healthy, you need to help your body maintain proper pH balance. Switching to a more alkaline-forming diet and confronting stress can go a long way toward preventing osteoporosis. You will learn more about stress-reducing lifestyle choices in chapter 7.

For more information on osteoporosis, consult my book *Healing Injuries the Natural Way*.

Weight Problems

According to biochemist Robert O. Young, yeasts and fungi contribute to both excessive thinness and obesity. That may sound contradictory, but to paraphrase Young's hypothesis, acidity caused by yeasts and fungi can cause excess weight to develop over time. In people with impaired natural body mechanisms, the result may be excessive thinness. Let me clarify: we already know that an overly acidic body encourages the overgrowth of yeasts and fungi, and that they, in turn, interfere with our digestion. Young states that excess weight can be caused not just by nutritional deficiencies but also by toxins in the colon that are the by-products of yeasts and fungi. The toxins enter the bloodstream through leaks in the lower bowel, and this poisoned blood travels to the liver. The Standard American Diet is already straining the liver, and the yeast and fungus toxins further compromise its ability to metabolize fat and sugar. Moreover, as one of the body's critical detoxification organs, the liver produces large amounts of LDL cholesterol (also known as "bad" cholesterol) to bind to toxins; if your other elimination systems are not functioning properly, this mixture gets stored in body tissue.[38]

In addition to yeasts and fungi, synthetic environmental and food toxins are linked with increased fat stores. Synthetic chemicals, such as industrial toxins and food preservatives, tend to be attracted to fat molecules as they move through the circulatory system, where they can cause tissue and organ damage, including damage to the brain. To prevent toxins from circulating, the body binds them to fat and holds on to its fat stores. For more information, consult my books *The Brain Wash* and *The 4-Week Ultimate Body Detox Plan*.

Acidic foods also play a significant role in weight gain. We tend to look at fat as the enemy, but fat is actually your ally against high levels of acidic food. This may sound counterintuitive, but bear with me as I explain. In the same way that your fat stores protect you from environmental toxins, they help to prevent acid from scouring your arteries and damaging your cells, tissues, and organs; ultimately, they save you from disease. Your body uses fat as a buffer against acid. If you keep eating highly acidic food or even moderately acidic food over a long period of time, without enough alkaline foods to counter the acidity, your body will pack on more and more fat in its effort to protect you from cell damage. Your body is, in effect, in preservation mode. You may hate the belly bulge, spare tire, and dimpled thighs, but those fat stores are saving your life.

If you're attempting to lose weight by following a high-protein diet such as Atkins or South Beach, you should know that these diets are pretty much a sure-fire way to unbalance your pH and make you vulnerable to disease. While they may help some people with short-term weight loss, they create an extreme state of acidity, and the rebound effect will ensure that you regain the weight you lost, and possibly more.

So forget the high-protein approach to weight loss and start kicking acid out of your body. Once it is alkalized, your body will no longer require its fat stores. By getting to the root cause of your weight gain rather than just trying to starve your body of energy, you'll eliminate excess weight and feel good at the same time. You won't suffer the jittery nerves or irritability of dieting. Instead, you'll be energized and less prone to illness, so you'll feel better than ever. You'll want to throw out the fad diets forever. The key to optimum weight is a balanced pH, which you can achieve through an alkaline diet and lifestyle choices. You'll learn more about both in the coming chapters.

You may be thinking, "Wait a minute. I know a skinny person who eats anything she wants and never gains weight." There are, indeed, many people who eat all kinds of acidic junk food and never pack on fat. I've known skinny people who were chain-smokers (thereby inhaling acidic toxins), junk food addicts, serious coffee drinkers, and loathers of all things vegetable. These people may seem relatively healthy, but their bodies are not working properly. An important protective mechanism (the fat buffering system) is malfunctioning. If acid is not adequately eliminated or buffered with fat, the body may start breaking down its own muscles, tissues, bones, and organs, which over time can lead to serious disease. Basically, being overweight and being underweight are two sides of the same coin: acidity.

If you are overweight, kicking acid out of your diet gives your body a chance to restore balance at the cellular level, which allows it to start breaking down fat stores and ultimately rebalance your weight. On the other side of the coin, if gaining weight is a struggle no matter how much food you eat, a more alkaline diet will help your body function properly and find a healthier weight.

pH Solution

Janine Overcomes Chronic Fatigue Syndrome

Janine, 33, a former women's clothing store manager, arrived at my office, assisted by her husband. The severe disabling symptoms of chronic fatigue syndrome had left her unable to work and barely able to walk. She had already "run the gamut" of health practitioners, both medical and holistic, and felt that she had "tried everything and nothing worked." I'm not a fan of such statements, as they are not only gross exaggerations but they also make a person feel further disempowered by their illness. I believe it's important to keep hope alive, no matter how much a person is suffering and even if other doctors have indicated that there is no hope. But I understood that Janine was overwhelmed by her fruitless quest for health improvement, so I gently reminded her that I had not yet had the opportunity to work with her. I told her I hoped she would give my approach a chance to work. She agreed to give it a try.

Having suffered for more than 15 years, Janine had initially been written off by medical doctors, who told her that her disabling fatigue, headaches, seemingly constant need for sleep or rest, and other symptoms were "all in her head." She later tried nutritionists, naturopaths, homeopaths, acupuncturists, massage therapists, and other holistic health practitioners. She had seen only minimal improvement over the years and had become discouraged by her lack of success in restoring her health.

For the first two weeks after starting the Kick Acid program, she didn't notice any improvements. But after the third week, Janine called to tell me that she'd gone for a long walk, at least by her standards. In a follow-up appointment a few months later, during which time she had strictly followed the Kick Acid program, Janine started crying tears of joy when she told me she had started to have days when her energy was substantially increased and she felt like she was back to her old self—the way she had felt before chronic fatigue syndrome. After only three months, she had experienced significant health improvements. She was still suffering some weakness and fatigue, but we anticipated even more improvements as her body continued to detoxify acid wastes and rebuild.

Janine is grateful that she tried this approach and has eliminated the words "tried everything" and "nothing worked" from her vocabulary. Now, whenever she hears someone say, "I've tried everything," she quickly responds, "You haven't tried kicking acid!"

CHAPTER 4

Making Wise Acid Choices

"Destiny is no matter of chance; it is a matter of choice. It is
not a thing to be waited for; it is a thing to be achieved."

—WILLIAM JENNINGS BRYAN

Healthy eating doesn't have to feel like punishment. You don't have to give up all of your favorite foods, eat like a rabbit, or live like a hermit. You can eliminate acidity in your body once and for all through simple food and lifestyle changes. The Ultimate pH Solution fits into any lifestyle, whether you're a stay-at-home parent, the CEO of a corporation, or a traveling salesperson. You can eat a more alkaline diet without feeling deprived. And you don't have to give up all acidic foods to feel great and prevent disease; you just need to make your body more alkaline to balance them out.

These four important steps will help you kick acid in your body for optimum health, healing, balanced weight, and disease prevention:

1. Eliminate harmful acidic foods from your diet.
2. Choose healthier acidic food options, and keep them at a low level in your diet—approximately 30 percent.
3. Increase alkaline foods to 70 percent of your diet.
4. Incorporate alkalizing lifestyle choices and alkalizing supplements into your life.

This chapter focuses on the first two steps, teaching you which acidic foods to avoid and which can be incorporated in moderation into a healthy diet. In chapter 5, you will learn which foods are alkalizing, and in chapters 6 and 7 you will learn about alkalizing supplements and lifestyle choices.

But before we get into which foods to add to or remove from your diet, let's discuss some of the many myths out there about balancing the body's pH.

DEBUNKING THE TOP 10 ACID MYTHS

If you've searched the Internet or read other books on the topic of pH balance, you've probably encountered conflicting information. For example, some sources list fruit as alkaline; others say it's acidic. There is so much inaccurate information about acidity and alkalinity in widespread circulation that you no doubt grew confused as you tried to sort through it all. Those who haven't read anything on this topic before now might be better off.

I've sifted through stacks of information and over a dozen books, sorting the facts from the rampant misinformation, to give you charts, food lists, and guidelines you can rely on. Along the way, I encountered some alarming myths:

1. **Some brands of coffee are alkaline; others are acidic.** All coffee is acidic, though brands that have been heavily sprayed with pesticides or processed with harmful chemicals may be more so. Sorry, folks. Other authors may try to placate their readers by misleading them, but I'd rather give you the facts so you can make better choices. Does that mean you need to swear off coffee? No. Just be aware that it is acid-forming and keep it to an absolute minimum. It's better as a treat than as a daily pick-me-up. A more alkaline diet will boost your energy in any case. (See Kick Acid Tip #4, on page 91, for natural, alkalizing energy boosters.)

2. **If you drink coffee on an empty stomach, or drink it black, it's alkalizing to the body.** I think coffee addicts repeat this myth to justify their habit. It doesn't matter whether you drink it on an empty stomach or a full one, and it doesn't matter whether you skip the sugar and cream (although these substances do add *more* acid). Coffee, once metabolized, has an acidic effect on your body. Period.

3. **Dairy products are alkalizing to the body.** In a laboratory, some dairy products may test alkaline, but, like other animal products, almost all dairy products are acid-forming once they're eaten (goat's milk is the exception).

4. **Lemons are very acidic in the body.** *Not true.* As you'll learn below, there is a difference between something that tests acidic on its own and something that has an acidic effect on the body. While lemons test acidic in a laboratory, once combined with your digestive juices and metabolized, they have an alkalizing effect and are an excellent way to rebalance your body. I recommend adding lemon juice to your drinking water and consuming it throughout the day (see Kick Acid Tip #1, on page 74).

5. **Tomatoes are acidic.** Tomatoes may seem acidic when you bite into them, but, like lemons, they have an alkalizing effect on the body. So feel free to enjoy a plate of spelt pasta (you'll learn more about this delicious ancient grain in the next chapter) topped with fresh tomato sauce.

6. **All protein foods are acidic.** We tend to think that meat is the only source of protein. Ask any vegetarian how many times they've been asked, "Where do you get your protein?" and you'll know how deeply embedded this myth is. All fruits and vegetables contain protein, as do grains, beans, and other foods. Almost all animal protein is acidic, but many vegetarian sources of protein are alkaline.

7. **Millet balances your pH.** I saw this one at a health food store, and it made me laugh. While it would be great if any food had the extraordinary ability to either alkalize your body when you're acidic or acidify it if, on some rare occasion, you became too alkaline, I'm sorry to tell you there's no such food. Millet, a tiny spherical grain, is slightly acidifying once eaten. However, it is full of fiber, vitamins, and minerals, so it is a healthy addition to a predominantly alkaline diet and a wise acid choice.

8. **Whole-grain bread is alkaline.** Very few types of bread are alkaline. Only a few grains have the potential to be alkalizing (you'll learn more about these grains in the next chapter). But bread made from these grains would still need to be devoid of yeast, shortening, butter, margarine, preservatives, rising agents, and white or wheat flour. Most store-bought bread is full of this junk and should be avoided. I've included some quick and easy bread recipes in chapter 8. You won't need a bread machine to prepare these delicious alkalizing breads, and you won't be spending your time kneading.

9. **All fruit is alkaline.** I wish this one was true, as I love most types of fruit. Unfortunately, most fruit is acidic. However, it is a healthy acidic food, and you can include it in your diet. A few types of fruit—lemons, limes, grapefruit (as long as it's not excessively sweet), tomatoes, and avocados—do have an alkalizing effect on your body.

10. **There's no difference between acidic and acid-forming foods.** Bear with me; this one can be a bit confusing. Foods and other substances can be tested in a laboratory prior to being ingested to determine whether they are alkaline or acidic, but that information is useless to a discussion about pH balance in the body because it doesn't take into account the biochemical reactions that occur during digestion. It is the interaction between a food and our digestive juices that determines whether the food has an overall alkalizing or acidifying effect on the body. Lemons, for example, test as

strongly acidic in a laboratory, but once ingested have an alkalizing effect.

To determine whether foods are acid- or alkaline-forming, researchers look at whether they have an acidic or alkaline ash when they are burned, since that is essentially what happens to food during the process of metabolism. The foods listed in this book as alkaline have all been tested for their effects on the body. It's irrelevant whether these foods test acid or alkaline on their own, and that information has the potential to be confusing, so I haven't included it.

KICK ACID TIP #1

Just Add Lemon

Every morning, I juice six lemons and pour the juice into a small jar to add to my alkaline water throughout the day. Fresh lemon juice supplies vitamin C and helps alkalize your body. And it is great for cleansing the liver. But you must use fresh lemons, not bottled lemon juice. If it's easier for you, juice the lemons the night before, so the juice is ready to take with you to work. This simple trick will go a long way toward alkalizing your body—and water with a fresh splash of lemon juice tastes great!

THE ALKALINE:ACID RATIO

The Ultimate pH Solution approach to great health and balanced weight is simple: strive to get a 70:30 ratio of alkaline food to acidic food. This is easier than you might think. You don't have to count calories and then calculate whether you ate the correct ratio. That's just not workable over the long term. All you have to do is estimate the ratio by the amounts of alkaline-forming foods on your plate at each meal or snack. You'll soon learn guidelines to help you remember which foods are acidic and which ones are alkaline, so you won't have to memorize massive food lists.

FREQUENTLY ASKED QUESTIONS

Q: Do I have to eliminate all acidic foods from my diet to follow the Kick Acid lifestyle?

A: You can still eat some acidic foods, although it's best to be selective and choose healthier acidic options. That doesn't mean you can never eat dessert or enjoy a steak dinner. However, pay attention to the effects these foods have on your pH; even an occasional "treat" can throw your balance off. You'll maintain a healthy pH balance by increasing your intake of alkaline foods to compensate for the acidic foods. Don't worry: you won't be counting grams of fat, carbs, or calories. This program is easy to start and to maintain for life. And, unlike fad diets, it's all about balance—and maintaining or achieving great health.

ELIMINATING HARMFUL ACIDIC FOODS FROM YOUR DIET

In chapter 1, you learned about the inherent problems with the Standard American Diet. And if you took the quiz in chapter 2, you now know how much of your food is acidic. We discussed the acid-forming nature of sugar, artificial food additives, rancid and trans fats, meat, dairy products, table salt, and soda. Some of these items, such as artificial food additives and trans fats, you would do well to avoid altogether; they have no redeeming qualities. They not only take the space of potentially healthier foods in our diets but are also linked to a lengthy list of diseases.

Not all acidic foods are created equal. Many fruits, for example, create acid in your body, but they also contribute beneficial nutrients, fiber, and phytonutrients (natural healing compounds found in plants). Soda, on the other hand, has nothing positive to contribute: it is full of colors, preservatives, sugar, and other unhealthy ingredients. While it's not necessary to eliminate all acid-forming foods from your diet, it's best to focus on eating the ones that actually do something good for you.

There are easy ways to cut back on acidic foods, and you'll usually find that you don't miss them as much as you thought you would. Let's start with sugar.

Kick the Sugar Habit

Sugar may taste sweet, but its health effects are anything but. Excessive sugar consumption throws our pH levels out of balance. The sugar and the acidity create

...t that is ripe for the overgrowth of dangerous yeasts, fungi, ...hese pathogens feed on the sugar, multiply, and expel toxic ...el even worse. Because they require more sugar to feed and ...get cravings for sweets, breads, pastas, and soda.

...is acidic, it is a far better option than sugary desserts. And stay clear of artificial sweeteners: not only are they highly acid-forming, they are also linked to many diseases. The only sweetener that isn't acid-forming is stevia, a naturally sweet herb. Use stevia instead of other sweeteners.

You were probably shocked to learn that the average person eats more than 150 pounds of sugar per year. While we typically eat a lot of sugar in the form of desserts and sugary beverages, a large portion of our sugar intake comes from hidden sources. Consider these seemingly unlikely sources of sugar:

- Livestock are often fed sugar prior to slaughter to improve the color and taste of the meat.
- Corn syrup and molasses are frequently used in restaurants to prevent shrinkage in hamburgers.
- Canned salmon is often glazed with sugar.
- Breading often contains sugar, as do bouillon cubes and dry-roasted nuts.
- Alcoholic beverages contain sugar.
- Condiments such as ketchup, mustard, relish, and many others are full of sugar.
- Familiar lunch and breakfast standbys such as luncheon meats, bacon, dry cereal, and peanut butter contain sugar.
- Table salt can contain sugar![1]
- The sports and "energy" drinks found in most health food or grocery stores contain plentiful amounts of sugar and tend to be extremely acid-forming, which can deplete your muscles of important minerals and counter some of the beneficial effects of exercise. Opt for a green drink instead.

The first step in kicking your sugar habit is to eliminate sources of sugar—hidden or not—from your diet, as well as foods that contribute to sugar cravings by lowering your blood sugar.

- Stop drinking soft drinks. You'll drastically cut down your sugar intake—by 11 teaspoons per can.
- Be wary of products that claim to contain "real fruit." They don't have to contain much to make that statement, and they likely contain "real sugar," and lots of it.

- Start reading labels! Any ingredient that ends in "-ose" is sugar. Some examples include glucose, galactose, mannose, and fructose.
- Better yet, stop buying packaged foods. Most packaged foods are loaded with sugar, synthetic food additives, and harmful fats. They are a sure-fire way to acidify your body.
- Avoid white flour products—breads, pasta, etc. Not only are these foods acid-forming, but the refined carbohydrates act like sugar in your body, causing blood sugar fluctuations that lead to sugar cravings. And white flour products typically contain sugar.
- Be wary of brown bread and "whole-grain" products—if it doesn't say "100% whole grain," it's probably predominantly white flour. As a better option, try one of the bread recipes in chapter 8.
- In addition to white flour and white sugar products, eliminate white potatoes and white rice. These foods are highly acid-forming and offer little or no nutritional value, yet they cause the same rapid blood sugar fluctuations as white sugar.
- Avoid coffee: it lowers your blood sugar and can trigger cravings for sweets.

There are a number of ways in which you can curb your sugar cravings:

- Start keeping track of all the foods you eat that contain sweeteners. When you learn how much sugar you are actually eating, you'll probably be motivated to cut back.
- Wean yourself off sweets over time. Eat them only in moderation and choose healthier options that are chemical-free and have not been "enriched" with nutrients. (See Kick Acid Tip #3, on page 89, for more information about "enriched products.")
- Avoid buying sweets—if they are not readily available when a craving comes, you'll be less likely to eat them.
- Think twice before reaching for sweets out of habit or in response to social pressures.
- Whenever you have a sugar craving, first drink a large glass of water (squeeze some fresh lemon juice into it for a great alkalizing and refreshing drink). Most people are chronically dehydrated and misinterpret the body's signals for water as cravings for food, especially sweets. If you drink water first, more often than not the craving for sweets will disappear.

If you're having trouble conquering your sugar cravings, there are many alternatives that will satisfy your sweet tooth. While some of these options can still increase the acidity of your body, they will be an improvement over mass consumption of refined white sugar.

- To sweeten dishes and baked goods, use a small amount of stevia, an herb that tastes 1,000 times sweeter than sugar yet doesn't cause the blood spikes and dips that sugar and other sweeteners do.
- Add sweet potatoes—cooked and mashed—to baked goods made with alkalizing grains.
- Use spices, such as cinnamon, cloves, and ginger, that have a natural sweetness to them.
- Have a piece of raw fruit. While most fruit is acidic, it is a substantially healthier option than refined sugar and foods made with it.
- When making fresh juices, add one apple if the taste is too bitter for you. You'll be amazed how good a glass of freshly juiced greens tastes when you add an apple to it. Apples are acidic, but their acidifying effects are balanced by the greens.
- Prepare the occasional sweet at home, using wholesome ingredients and limited amounts of sweeteners. For ideas, turn to chapter 8. You can whip up delicious chocolate mousse in less than 5 minutes.

KICK ACID TIP #2

Cut Out Cola and Other Sodas

Kick the soda habit and you'll be well on your way to kicking acid in your body. Cola rates between 2.52 and 2.61 on the pH scale. Also, it forms an overwhelming amount of acid in your body—acid that must be neutralized with valuable minerals and water. Remember that you need to drink 32 cups of water (and expend tremendous amounts of energy that would be better used elsewhere in your body) just to neutralize the acidity of one glass of soda. Skip the soda and you'll have more energy and water available for healing your body and cleansing your cells and tissues.

Forgo Faux Food

Not even the food industry would dare claim that synthetic colors, flavors, preservatives, and other food additives are healthy. But their dirty little secret is that many of these ingredients can actually damage your health. More and more research shows that, in addition to being acid-forming, many of these additives have neurotoxic effects, meaning they are harmful to the brain and nervous system.

There are a number of easy ways to eliminate harmful food additives from your diet:

- Avoid processed, packaged, or prepared foods. Instead, think fresh— fresh produce, that is!
- Eat organic as much as possible. Fruit, vegetables, grains, and other foods tend to be heavily sprayed. By choosing organic food, you'll reduce your exposure to acid-forming and toxic pesticide residues.
- Avoid products that claim to be "sugar-free" or "no sugar added"—they typically contain artificial sweeteners. Don't be tricked by companies claiming that their products travel through the digestive tract untouched or unabsorbed. The only such products are those that are not recognized as food by your body. Sugar, while far from perfect, is a better option than a chemical sweetener.
- Avoid fast-food restaurants: they use harmful additives such as MSG, stabilizers, trans fats, preservatives, fillers, and other ingredients that are potentially harmful to your body.
- Read labels. If you spot any ingredients that you don't recognize and can barely pronounce, avoid the product. Real food doesn't need a lengthy ingredient list, nor does it include FD&C Yellow No. 5, sodium benzoate, polysorbate 80, or monosodium glutamate. Kick foods with chemical additives right out of your diet.

Say Sayonara to Table Salt

Table salt, the most commonly used type of salt, is acid-forming. I recommend that you switch to Celtic sea salt or Himalayan salt, which are alkalizing to the body. Celtic sea salt and similar unrefined sea salts look gray and a bit moist. Himalayan salt has a naturally occurring orange color. Both types of salt contain a healthier, alkalizing form of sodium and are packed with many other minerals, including potassium and calcium.

While these alternatives are better for you than white salt, it's still important to reduce your salt intake and acquaint yourself with the natural, subtler flavors of food. We've become accustomed to the taste of excessively salted foods, which tend to dehydrate our bodies and unbalance our electrolytes. Switching to Celtic sea salt or Himalayan salt is a good start, but don't use these options to excess either. Your taste buds will adjust over time.

Banish Unhealthy Fats

It's essential to eliminate unhealthy, acid-forming fats from your diet. You learned about the harmful effects of trans fats in chapter 1. Read the labels on packages and avoid anything with trans fats, hydrogenated fats, or partially hydrogenated fats. You'll find this information in the Nutrition Facts table or the ingredient list.

Stay away from margarine. And be aware that packaged baked goods, as well as those from traditional bakeries, typically contain either margarine or another hydrogenated fat, such as shortening.

Avoid fried foods. If you crave french fries, opt for a baked sweet potato instead. Or try my recipe for Yam Fries on page 167. They taste great and are nutritious too. French fries can't compete with that.

Minimize Meat Consumption

Almost all animal products are highly acid-forming, including beef, veal, pork, bacon, luncheon meats, eggs, milk, cheese, organ meats, poultry, farm-raised fish, and shellfish. Cut back on your consumption of these foods and it will be easier to tip the pH scales in your favor. Don't worry about getting enough protein; there are many great sources of protein that are healthier alternatives than meat and dairy. Vegetarian options include bean sprouts, alfalfa sprouts, tofu, lentils, legumes (chickpeas, navy beans, pinto beans, kidney beans), pumpkin seeds, almonds, and avocados. Even spinach, broccoli, green leaf lettuce, kale, peas, zucchini, carrots, lemons, garlic, and blueberries contain some protein.

Pound for pound, many vegetables and legumes have a higher protein-calorie percentage than meat. Avocados contain more usable protein than an 8-ounce steak—and healthy fatty acids too. No steak can make that claim. Not all vegetables and legumes are alkaline, but they are loaded with fiber and other nutrients and are a healthier option than most types of meat. And none of these protein sources contains the steroids, antibiotics, hormones, and saturated fats found in most of the meat supply.

Current research has debunked the myth that we need high levels of protein in our diet. In the past 200 years, we have seen the experts reduce the recommended daily amount from more than 100 grams to 60 grams, and some experts believe the ideal amount to be less than 30 grams. The human body is designed to obtain its protein requirements from vegetables, nuts, seeds, and legumes. You can still have meat occasionally if you wish; just remember that it is highly acid-forming and eat more alkaline foods to compensate.

Do Away with Dairy Products

There are many great alternatives to milk, such as almond milk, rice milk, and soy milk. They don't have the same taste as cow's milk, but each has its own unique flavor. They can be substituted in recipes or drunk in place of cow's milk. Almond milk and soy milk are alkaline-forming; however, if they are sweetened, the sugar can offset the alkalizing effects, so look for the unsweetened kind. Or try my recipe for delicious, creamy Almond Milk, on page 145.

As for cheese, most of the substitutes on the market contain milk protein from cow's milk (called casein), among other acidifying ingredients. Even some of the dairy-free options are acidifying, thanks to the many unhealthy ingredients used, including trans fats, hydrogenated fats, and other additives. It's best to avoid cheese and cheese substitutes altogether.

Skip butter as well, as it is acidic. Opt instead for Michelle's Better Butter (page 154), a quick and simple butter alternative made with healthy oils. It tastes great! You can keep it in the fridge to spread on anything you would normally use butter on.

Abandon Alcohol

Alcoholic beverages of all kinds, including those claiming to use alkaline water, are highly acid-forming in your body. Alcohol supports the proliferation of harmful bacteria and viruses. In addition to alcohol's high sugar content and addictive, potentially health-damaging properties, the ethanol in alcohol is converted by the liver into acetaldehyde, which is the toxic compound linked to hangovers. (Acetaldehyde is also a by-product of car emissions, tobacco smoke, and industrial processes.) While acetaldehyde also occurs in trace amounts in ripe fruit, coffee, and bread, alcoholic beverages contain amounts that are unhealthy for the body to handle.

It's best to cut out alcohol altogether, but remember, the Ultimate pH Solution is intended to be a lifestyle you can live with. If you can't imagine life without an occasional beer or glass of wine, just watch the rest of your diet on those days. Do try to keep your intake of alcoholic beverages to a minimum.

THE TRUTH ABOUT CRAVINGS

Cravings are your body's way of letting you know that something is missing from your diet. We often reach for sugary desserts, potato chips, or soda because we can't bear the cravings or don't understand what they mean. But most food cravings are your body's way of letting you know that you are dehydrated and need more pure water. Because most people are accustomed to overeating, we just assume that we need more food.

If you're craving acid-forming junk food, you're probably dehydrated. Before rushing out for chips or a chocolate bar, drink a large glass of pure water with the juice of half a lemon squeezed into it. Most cravings will be eliminated in a matter of minutes. If your craving doesn't disappear, it may be a sign that you have a vitamin or mineral deficiency. That's why no amount of junk food tends to satisfy cravings. Your body needs wholesome, healthy foods full of vitamins and minerals. As you change your diet to include more alkalizing foods, your cravings will disappear. If you still experience them, add more variety to your diet and drink more alkaline water.

The Kick Acid Hit List

The foods in the following table share one common thread: they're all acidic. While this list is by no means complete, it shows some of the most common acidifying foods you may be eating. Refer to it as often as necessary to help you kick acid. The list may look long, but don't worry: I won't leave you feeling deprived. You'll soon learn about healthy acidic foods you *can* include in your diet (in moderation), and in the next chapter, we'll talk about the many alkalizing foods you can eat in plentiful amounts.

COMMON ACIDIC FOODS TO ELIMINATE OR REDU

Dairy Products	Meat, Poultry and Fish*	Vegetables	Fruit	
Milk	Beef	Mushrooms	Canned fruit of	White flour
Cream	Veal	White potatoes	all kinds	Baked goods of
Hard cheese	Pork		Pickled fruit	all kinds that
Cottage cheese	Organ meats		Fruit syrups	contain white
Ice cream	Poultry		Jam	flour
Yogurt	Eggs		Jelly	White bread
Most soy	Shellfish		Pie filling	Multigrain
cheeses	Farmed fish			bread made
Goat's milk				with white
cheese				flour
Whey				Rye bread
Casein (and all				made with
foods that				white flour
contain this				Whole wheat
acidic milk				bread or pasta
protein)				Whole-grain
				bread
				White rice

Nuts and Seeds	Extras	Fats and Oils	Sweeteners	Beverages
Salted nuts of	Ketchup	Margarine	White sugar	Alcohol
all kinds	Mayonnaise	Butter	Refined sugar	(including
Unrefrigerated	Mustard	Clarified butter	Brown sugar	beer and
nuts	Vinegar	(ghee)	Turbinado sugar	wine)
Most packaged	Soy sauce	Corn oil	Fructose	Fruit juice,
nuts	Yeast		Corn syrup	sweetened
	Malt		Honey,	
	Table salt		pasteurized	
	MSG			

* This list refers to non-organic meat, which is not only highly acidic but tends to contain many toxins, such as pesticide residues, hormones, and antibiotics. Organic meat contains fewer harmful toxins but is still acid-forming; it is best to keep it to a minimum in your diet or avoid altogether.

HEALTHIER ACID OPTIONS

Not all acidic foods should be eliminated from your diet. Remember, your body shouldn't be too acidic *or* too alkaline; it is important to find balance. Choose healthier acidic food options and keep them to about 30 percent of your diet.

The Healing Power of Fruit

It's hard to argue the value of fresh fruit. Most fruit is packed with life-sustaining nutrients and natural phytochemicals—plant chemicals that have medicinal properties. The majority, however, contain a significant amount of sugar. Many people aren't aware that modern agricultural science and bio-technology have tampered with fruit crops to breed species with increased sugar content. This disturbing side of food science has also increased the average size of apples, oranges, and other fruits so that a serving is larger today than it was a century ago.

If you have a sugar craving, fresh fruit is generally the best way to satisfy it. The sugar in fruit can contribute to an acid condition in the body, but fruit at least has immense nutritional value, unlike most other acidic choices. The Standard American Diet is heavy on processed foods, which have a high sugar content. Most people are drunk on sugar well before they eat a piece of fruit. Add in some complex carbohydrates, which also break down into sugar in the digestive tract, and you get a sense of the disturbing amount of acidity sugar alone will cause.

That being said, the typical North American does not eat enough fresh fruit. Instead, we consume fruit juice (which often contains no actual fruit juice at all), processed fruit cups, canned fruit, and fruit pie fillings, most of which have large amounts of sugar added. I had the great pleasure of speaking with Harvey Diamond, the renowned author of the bestselling book *Fit for Life*. He spoke openly about the disturbing trend in which people readily eat candy bars and drink soda but don't consider fruit part of a healthy diet. He remarked on the thousands of medicinal phytochemicals found in fruit, then laughed and added, "When was the last time you heard about a new miracle substance in pork chops?" And he's right. The vast majority of substances that protect your body from disease are found in fresh fruits and vegetables.

Berries are some of the healthiest fruits. Blueberries, raspberries, and straw-berries contain plentiful amounts of polyphenols, natural substances that prevent oxidative damage in the blood, brain, and tissues. Blueberries were one of the top antioxidant foods tested by the U.S. Department of Agriculture (USDA). Research shows that by eating blueberries regularly you can stop the decline of heat-shock proteins, compounds that are critical to brain health yet decrease as people age, resulting in brain inflammation and damage.[2] A study of rats fed extracts of blueberries (along with strawberry and spinach extracts) showed that the potent antioxidants actually *reversed* some of the effects of age-related brain decline.[3] Blueberries also contain a substance that is 10 times more effective than Aspirin at reducing both pain and inflammation. Blueberries are true superfoods that should be eaten regularly and are a delicious alternative to unhealthy sweets. While berries, blueberries included, are acid-forming in the body, they have so many health merits that they should be a regular part of the 30 percent healthy acidic foods in your diet.

While most fruit is acidic, several, such as lemons, limes, grapefruit, tomatoes, and avocados, are alkaline-forming. (Yes, the latter two foods are actually fruit.) You'll be amazed at some of the more unconventional uses for avocado, such as Chocolate Mousse (page 171). If you're not a fan of avocado, don't worry: you won't even know you're eating it (and neither will your kids if you decide to share this delicious dessert with them). My parents couldn't stand avocado until I suggested they try my chocolate mousse. Now they're hooked.

Wonders of the Sea

The omega-3 fatty acids found in fish and fish oil are one of nature's weapons against brain diseases such as Alzheimer's and depression, pain disorders, and immune system malfunctions. In one study, researchers genetically engineered mice to develop Alzheimer's. The mice were divided into two groups: one group was fed a diet rich in docosahexanoic acid (DHA), the type of omega-3 fatty acid found in cold-water fish; the other group was fed a diet low in DHA. In only five months, researchers found 70 percent less amyloid protein—the plaque implicated in Alzheimer's disease—in mice fed the high-DHA diet. The same group of researchers had previously found that DHA enabled mice to perform better on memory tests.[4]

Mice are not the only ones who can benefit from fish oils. DHA makes up a large part of the lining of our brain cells, so it is imperative to eat a diet rich in these omega-3 fats to keep the cellular lining flexible enough to allow memory messages to pass between cells. DHA promotes nerve transmission in the central nervous system and protects the energy centers of the cells—the mitochondria—from damage. That ensures better brain health and better health for the rest of our body as well, since mitochondria provide energy for most of our bodily functions.

So while fish is acid-forming in our bodies, it offers such tremendous health benefits that it is a wise acid choice. The Ultimate pH Solution is all about maximizing great health, and fish can play an important role to that end. Just be sure to choose fish that contain high amounts of omega-3 fatty acids, such as mackerel, sardines, salmon, lake trout, and herring. But be aware that some fatty cold-water fish have become contaminated with heavy metals and other toxins, and avoid fish that consistently show up high on the mercury radar, including predatory fish such as swordfish and shark, as well as sea bass, northern pike, tuna, walleye, and largemouth bass. Salmon raised in fish farms also frequently shows up with high amounts of mercury, and it often contains antibiotic residues and has lower levels of the important omega-3 fatty acids. To avoid the toxins, always choose wild salmon over farmed salmon.

If you can't stand the thought of fish, you can take fish oil supplements instead.

ESSENTIAL FATTY ACIDS

The human body produces all the fatty acids it needs, with the exception of linoleic acid (an omega-6 fatty acid) and alpha-linolenic acid (an omega-3 fatty acid). We require omega-3 and omega-6 essential fatty acids (EFAs) to produce the fats needed for protection of cell membranes, joint lubrication, energy production, and a host of other critical functions. Omega-3 fatty acids are found in certain seed oils (such as hemp, flax, walnut, and soybean), as well as in cold-water fish. Omega-6 EFAs are found in flaxseed oil, sunflower seeds, and lesser-known seed sources such as black currant, evening primrose, and borage.[5]

Omega-3 EFAs are beneficial in many ways: they keep our blood from getting too sticky; they reduce inflammation; and they help lower blood pressure and triglyceride levels (which are implicated in many cardiovascular diseases). Omega-6 EFAs help lower blood pressure and blood cholesterol levels, reducing the risk of stroke and heart disease. They improve fat metabolism in people with diabetes and can alleviate arthritis. They increase the metabolic rate, which may lead to weight loss and fat reduction. They are also effective at relieving symptoms of premenstrual syndrome and are good for your hair, skin, and nerves.[6]

Many foods, such as cereals, vegetable oils, eggs, and poultry, are sources of these fatty acids; however, most of these foods are acid-forming and should be eaten in the 30 percent portion of your diet. Alkaline sources of EFAs include flaxseeds, flaxseed oil, hemp seeds, hempseed oil, olive oil, avocados, and other oils, nuts, and seeds listed in the Kick Acid Hot List (page 97).

The Whole Grain and Nothing But the Grain

Not all grains were created equal. This is especially true when you're trying to balance your body chemistry. Most grains are acid-forming, especially white flour and whole wheat flour. Barley, corn, rye, and oat bran (the fibrous part of the oat) are also extremely acid-forming and are best avoided or eaten in small amounts. Like white flour, white rice should be avoided, as it has very little nutritional value.

There are varying degrees of wise acid choices. Brown rice, wild rice, and oats are only moderately acid-forming and can be part of the 30 percent acidic portion of your diet. Brown rice offers vitamin E and is high in fiber. Wild rice (which is not truly a grain but a seed) is high in protein, fiber, B vitamins, and potassium. Oats stabilize blood sugar, lower cholesterol, and are high in protein and fiber. Oats are available as instant, steel-cut, rolled, bran, groats, flakes, and flour. Avoid instant oats that contain sugar.

Amaranth, kasha, millet, and triticale are even better, less acid-forming choices. Amaranth is an ancient grain that has a nutty flavor and is loaded with protein, lysine, calcium, iron, potassium, and magnesium. It can be ground into flour for use in breads, noodles, pancakes, or baked goods. Kasha is another name for buckwheat when it is roasted in its whole-grain state—in other words, not cut into groats or ground into flour. Whole-grain kasha may be cooked as a main dish or side dish, added to soups or casseroles, or ground into flour for breads, muffins, or pancakes. Millet is rich in protein and is only mildly acidic when eaten. It can replace rice in recipes or can be eaten as a hot breakfast cereal. Triticale is a hybrid of wheat and rye but is less acidic and substantially more nutritious than either. Packed with protein, fiber, and vitamin E, triticale can be cooked as a whole grain or ground into flour, which is available preground from many health food stores. See the cooking chart on page 172 for instructions on cooking these grains.

Your best whole-grain options are quinoa, buckwheat groats, and spelt. You'll learn more about these alkaline-forming grains in chapter 5, where we'll discuss the many great foods that will form the bulk of your food choices on the Kick Acid program.

WISE ACID FOODS THAT CAN BE EATEN AS PART OF A HEALTHY DIET

"Dairy" Products	Meat, Poultry, and Fish*	Legumes	Fruit	Grains
Rice milk, unsweetened Soy milk, unsweetened Vegan soy cheese (made without casein, sweeteners, preservatives, hydrogenated fats, or trans fats)	Beef, organic Organ meats, organic Poultry, organic Eggs, organic Freshwater fish (wild only, not farmed) Ocean fish (wild only, not farmed)	Black beans Chickpeas (garbanzo beans) Kidney beans	Apples Apricots Bananas Berries Cantaloupe Cherries (sweet) Currants Dates (fresh) Figs (fresh) Grapes Guava Honeydew melon Mangos Nectarines Oranges Papaya Peaches Persimmons Pineapple Plums Tangerines Watermelon Dried fruit, organic (without sulfites)*	Amaranth Barley Brown rice Kasha Millet Oatmeal Oats or oat bran Rye* Triticale Wild rice

Nuts and Seeds**	Extras	Oils	Sweeteners	Beverages
Brazil nuts Cashews Hazelnuts Peanuts Pecans Pistachios Walnuts Flaxseeds Sunflower seeds	Carob, organic, unsweetened Cocoa, organic, unsweetened Curry powder Nutmeg Vanilla	Canola oil (organic, cold-pressed, GMO-free) Grapeseed oil Sunflower oil	Barley malt syrup Brown rice syrup Cane juice Honey, unpasteurized Maple syrup Sugarcane, organic, unrefined	Black or green tea* Fruit juice, unsweetened, with no preservatives, additives, or colors

* Highly acidic; eat occasionally in small amounts or avoid altogether.
** With the exception of flaxseeds and sunflower seeds, all nuts and seeds should be fresh, raw, unsalted, and refrigerated.

KICK ACID TIP #3

Avoid "Enriched" Foods

When I was writing an article for a women's magazine, I had the good fortune to discuss "enriched" foods with author Dana Carpender. While we have different philosophies about healthy eating, she is a vibrant and funny woman, and she shared a great analogy with me. She tells people that enriched flour products are "typically grain products that have had all the fiber and some 35 or more nutrients removed and five added back in. Enriched flour products are comparable to being robbed of all your clothes, money, shoes, and personal belongings while walking to the bus stop. Then the thief gives you your shoes and a quarter for the bus and tells you that you've been 'enriched' by the experience. Not likely."

So-called enriched products are misleading and unhealthy. Avoid them altogether. That includes the new "vitamin-enriched sparkling beverages"—a fancy name to market soda. Don't be fooled by marketing gimmicks. Contrary to what the food processing giants tell you, your health certainly won't be enriched by these products.

pH Solution
Barbara Beats Fibromyalgia

Barbara was referred to me after she heard about my success with a fellow fibromyalgia sufferer. A tall, refined woman in her 60s, Barbara was experiencing the low energy, extreme pain, poor sleep, and general weariness that affects many people with debilitating fibromyalgia. What's more, Barbara had been living with these symptoms for what she described as "forever!"

After reviewing her health history, I learned that Barbara ate a largely acidic diet, even though she described it as "very healthy." Typical choices included chicken, fish, low-fat yogurt, whole wheat bread, milk, baked potatoes, and a green or orange vegetable or two at every meal. Like many others following a moderate- to high-protein diet, she was increasing the acidity of her blood, and therefore that of her tissues, without realizing it.

The acidic tissues spelled P-A-I-N for Barbara, which she rated as a 10 on a scale of 0 to 10 (10 being the worst pain she'd ever experienced). Barbara told me she had stopped doing many of the things she loved—hiking, cycling, traveling. She found exercising difficult because of the fatigue and pain. She often woke in the night, her body racked with pain, and her sleep deficit continued to grow.

I asked her to minimize the acidic foods she was eating, completely avoid dairy products and meat, and start eating an alkaline diet with lots more vegetables, legumes, and soy. I told her she could continue eating fish twice a week because, while fish is acidic, it offers beneficial omega-3 fatty acids that are deficient in most people with fibromyalgia. I also explained that the backlog of toxins in her tissues was contributing to her pain and fatigue, and that fruit, while acidic, has superb cleansing effects. She should eat fruit every morning on an empty stomach to maximize detoxification. Because cleansing is so important in the treatment of fibromyalgia, she should also drink at least 12 cups of pure water with fresh lemon juice a day, including first thing in the morning.

At her follow-up appointment one month later, Barbara told me she'd experienced huge improvements. She'd had trouble giving up dairy products, but felt that the overwhelmingly positive changes in her health made it worth the effort. I asked her again to rate her pain on a scale of 0 to 10. She laughed and said, "No, you don't understand. When I said I had experienced huge improvements, I meant that I don't have any pain anymore."

What's more, she told me, her energy was better than ever and her sleep had improved. She had started hiking again and was participating in cycling competitions and taking belly-dancing classes. She was doing things that many people half her age couldn't do! Barbara felt like a new woman and was even challenging her grandchildren to join her in her activities.

CHAPTER 5

Alkalizing for Lasting Health

"Once you make a decision, the universe conspires to make it happen."

—RALPH WALDO EMERSON

Now that you know which acidic foods to avoid and which wise acid choices are suited for about 30 percent of your diet, you're probably wondering what foods are left for the remaining 70 percent. In this chapter, you'll learn about the foods on the opposite side of the pH spectrum—alkaline foods—and some basic rules of thumb to help you remember them so you can make them a regular part of your diet. You'll find out how to prepare foods for maximum alkalizing effect and even how to continue eating some of your favorites while still nixing acid! At the end of this chapter, there's a table of the acid–alkaline spectrum to show you that there are varying degrees of acidity and alkalinity even in the healthiest foods.

KICK ACID TIP #4

Enjoy Natural, Alkalizing Energy Boosters

There are so many great natural energy boosters that you'll never need to rely on acid-forming coffee for an artificial boost of nervous energy. Instead, try these quick pick-me-ups:

- **Peppermint herbal tea:** The natural essential oils found in peppermint are proven to lift energy and moods—plus, it tastes great. Add a few drops of stevia for a sweeter tea.
- **Green drink:** Blend a teaspoon of a green powder supplement into a large glass of water. There are many different kinds, typically made from barley grass,

wheatgrass, alfalfa, spirulina, or another type of concentrated green plant. Don't let the color or the "green" name intimidate you; most green powders are naturally sweet and have a pleasant taste. Even better, they are packed with alkalizing nutrients that give your brain and body a boost. Drink two to four glasses per day for plenty of energy and alkalizing power all day long.

- **Yerba maté tea:** Known as the "ancient drink of health and friendship," yerba maté is a plant that grows in South America. Instead of caffeine, it contains mateine, which offers a healthy energy boost without jitteriness, plus the benefits of magnesium and potassium. It has even been shown to exhibit significant cancer-fighting properties.[1] It has a strong herbal taste, which may take some time to get used to. I enjoy yerba maté combined with peppermint herbal tea and a few drops of stevia for a great-tasting, natural pick-me-up.
- **Lemon water:** Pour yourself a large glass of pure, alkaline water and add the juice of a whole fresh lemon. This is a great energy booster that helps lessen pain and improve immunity by going to the source of these problems—excess acidity. If this is too tart for your taste, quickly turn it into lemonade with a few drops of stevia.
- **Pure peppermint essential oil:** In research, peppermint oil has been shown to provide a quick boost of energy when inhaled. Put a few drops of the oil on a handkerchief and inhale, or add a few drops to an aromatherapy diffuser and breathe deeply. Make sure you're using pure peppermint essential oil and not "fragrance" oil, which is synthetic and usually contains toxic ingredients.

ALKALINE FOODS

There are many delicious alkaline foods you can eat, including most vegetables, some grains and legumes, and a few fruits. There are even great alkaline alternatives to many of your favorite acidic foods. Following the Ultimate pH Solution is not about starvation or deprivation, it's about learning a new way to eat and live in harmony with your body for fantastic health. Once you start giving your body what it needs to feel great, you will find that cravings for junk food and sweets disappear. Many people even start craving healthier options. I always know when I'm not getting enough greens in my diet because I start craving salads. I would have never guessed that anyone would crave salads, but I do.

The Veggie Solution

Virtually all vegetables, with the exception of potatoes, are alkalizing to your body. Unlike white or red potatoes, sweet potatoes and yams are alkaline-forming, as are leafy greens, carrots, and even tomatoes. Knowing that, it is easy to eat a more alkalizing diet: a simple way to make every meal more alkaline-forming is to focus on vegetables instead of meat or grains. In chapter 8, you'll find more than 50 recipes for great vegetable-based foods, such as Red Pepper–Butternut Squash Quesadillas (page 163), Yam Fries (page 167), Tuna-less Salad Sandwiches (page 165), and many more. Even the most die-hard meat lover can learn to enjoy vegetables. Just ask my husband: he is proof that even a meat-and-potatoes man can love the Kick Acid program.

When incorporating vegetables into your diet, try spending a little more time in the produce department of your grocery store to find options you've never considered. Don't be afraid to ask questions. I've learned about some great exotic fruits and vegetables by asking grocery store employees what something is and how to use it.

KICK ACID TIP #5

Boost Your Brain Power with Avocado

Healthy fatty acids like those found in avocados help protect the brain and nervous system from damage. Our brains are 60 percent fat, which needs to be replenished to build healthy brain cells. Avocados also contain more usable protein than an 8-ounce steak. They are alkalizing in the body and help regulate your blood's biochemistry. They make a great addition to salads, can be used to garnish chili or wraps, and can even be the key ingredient in chocolate or berry mousse. See chapter 8 for more recipe ideas.

Wonder Grains

As we discussed in the previous chapter, most grains create acidity in your body. The exceptions are buckwheat groats, spelt, and quinoa, which are slightly alkalizing. Spelt is an ancient grain that, while part of the wheat family, is not acid-forming like wheat. Some people with wheat allergies can tolerate spelt. Also, spelt has a substantially higher nutritional value than whole wheat. Quinoa—a staple of the ancient Incas, who revered it as sacred—is not a true grain; rather, it is an herb. It is a complete protein and is high in iron, B vitamins, and fiber.

Beans, Beans, the Magical Fruit

Okay, beans are not fruit at all. They are legumes, a class of vegetables that includes beans, peas, and lentils. While some legumes are slightly acidifying, others are alkalizing in the body. Regardless, they are nutrition powerhouses that are worth adding to your diet. They are usually low in fat and high in protein, folate (vitamin B$_9$), potassium, iron, and magnesium. They also contain phytochemicals, a group of compounds that help to prevent chronic diseases such as cancer and heart disease, among others. As if that weren't enough, they're loaded with fiber, which helps eliminate toxins from your body through your bowels. Eating a diet high in fiber can reduce your risk of developing heart disease and diabetes.

Alkalizing legumes include lima beans, navy beans, soybeans, and lentils. You can eat other types of legumes as part of the 30 percent wise acid choices. The alkalizing legumes can be eaten as part of the 70 percent alkaline options.

The Joy of Soy

Soy products are alkalizing in varying degrees, depending on whether you are eating soy nuts, edamame (green soybeans), tofu, or soy flour. Soy nuts are highly alkaline; edamame (pronounced ed-dah-MAH-meh) are moderately alkaline; tofu and soy flour are slightly alkaline. All of these products contain isoflavones, plant-based compounds that may reduce the risk of some types of cancer. They are an excellent part of the 70 percent alkaline portion of your diet. Because all of these soy products are alkalizing to your body, there's no need to memorize *how* alkalizing they are. I've just provided the information for your interest.

Soy lecithin, a component of soy that consists of the nutrient phosphatidylcholine and essential fatty acids, is also alkalizing, which is great because it can be added to blended drinks for added nutritional value. Lecithin helps regulate blood pressure and protect the brain from toxins and the liver from fatty buildup.

Avoid desserts, ice cream, and meat alternatives made from soy. These products usually include acidic ingredients such as sugar, hydrogenated fats, or wheat gluten.

The Kick Acid Hot List

Because so much of the Western diet is acidic, it is virtually impossible to eat too many alkaline foods. You'll be amazed at how easy it can be to make alkaline foods 70 percent of your diet. On the next two pages is a list of alkaline foods to help you get started. Don't worry about memorizing it: you'll soon catch on to this new way of eating. I encourage people to keep copies of this list in their wallet or purse and on the fridge. You can assume that most items not on the list are acidic and should either be excluded from your diet or eaten as part of the 30 percent acidic foods.

To obtain maximum nutritional value and alkalizing power from your foods, try to eat organic foods as much as possible. Research comparing organic produce to traditionally farmed produce regularly shows substantially higher vitamin and mineral content in organic foods. Also, organic foods are free of acid-forming toxic pesticides and genetically modified ingredients.

EATING THE KICK ACID WAY

The way you prepare food is as important to good health as the foods you choose, and there are lots of great ways to use the delicious alkaline foods on the Kick Acid Hot List. Some of them may be new to your repertoire, but an experimental spirit is all you need to figure out how to incorporate them into your life. To get you started, I've offered some advice and suggestions over the next few pages, and the recipes in chapter 8 will give you even more ideas.

Using Cooking Oils

Never allow oil to get so hot it smokes. The temperature at which an oil will smoke varies from one type to another. The smoke temperature is the point at which the heat chemically alters the oil. If your cooking oil smokes, throw it out and start again. It is far better to use a lower temperature when cooking with oils and take a few extra minutes than to destroy the health properties of the meal by overheating it. Olive oil is a good choice for sautéing foods, as it can withstand temperatures up to about 325°F. Coconut oil can handle temperatures up to 350°F.

The source of the oil determines how acidic or alkaline the oil will be. Soy, coconut, olive, and almond oils are typically alkaline, while corn, canola,

O EAT IN PLENTIFUL AMOUNTS

	gumes	Fruit	Grains
Beets	amame (green soybeans)	Avocados	Buckwheat groats
Broccoli	entils	Cherries (sour)	Quinoa
Brussels sprouts	Lima beans	Coconut (fresh, unsweetened)	Spelt
Cabbage	Soy flour	Grapefruit (preferably not too sweet)	
Carrots	Soy lecithin	Lemons	
Cauliflower	Soy nuts	Limes	
Celery	Tofu	Tomatoes	
Chives	White navy beans		
Collard greens			
Comfrey			
Cucumbers			
Dandelion greens			
Endive			
Garlic			
Gingerroot			
Green beans			
Horseradish (fresh)			
Kale			
Kohlrabi			
Leeks			
Lettuce			
Mustard greens			
Okra			
Onions			
Peas			
Peppers, bell			
Peppers, hot (fresh, not pickled)			
Radishes			
Rhubarb			
Rutabaga			
Sea vegetables (such as agar, arame, dulse, hijiki, and nori)			
Sorrel			
Soy sprouts			
Spinach			
Sprouts			
Sweet potatoes			
Turnips			
Watercress			
Yams			
Zucchini			

Nuts and Seeds	Herbs and Spices	Oils	Beverages
Almond milk (unsweetened or sweetened with stevia) Almonds Caraway seeds Cumin seeds Fennel seeds Pumpkin seeds Sesame seeds Sprouted seeds (e.g., alfalfa, red clover, or broccoli)	Most herbs and spices (the exceptions are curry powder, nutmeg, and vanilla) Celtic sea salt Himalayan salt Cayenne pepper Red pepper flakes	Avocado oil Borage oil Coconut oil Cod liver oil Evening primrose oil Flaxseed oil Marine lipids Olive oil	Alkaline water Fresh vegetable juice

walnut, and sunflower oils are acidic. For more information, see the Alkaline–Acid Food Table, on page 177. You don't have to forgo all acidic oils; just remember that they should be eaten in moderation as part of your 30 percent wise acid choices.

Raw Power

Try to eat at least some raw fruits and vegetables every day. Raw foods, or foods cooked at temperatures lower than 118°F, contain plentiful amounts of natural enzymes, which help your digestion, thereby maximizing the nutrients absorbed. When you eat foods in their raw state, your body will not need to use as many of its own digestive enzymes, which frees up energy for healing processes. Enzymes also work like miniature Pac-Men in your body, eating up free radicals, reducing inflammation, and cleaning up your blood and tissues.

I'm not referring to raw meat when I encourage you to eat raw foods. While traditional cultures such as the Inuit in northern Canada have eaten meat raw as soon as it is caught, it is rare to find animal foods that fresh in grocery stores. Meat is prone to spoilage via bacteria and other microbes that start breaking it down soon after it has been caught or slaughtered. These microscopic pathogens may not be visible, but they are dangerous. Do not eat raw meat on the Kick Acid program. Sushi or sashimi, prepared by a skilled, reputable chef who uses the freshest fish possible, can be an occasional exception.

KICK ACID TIP #6

Eat a Large Salad Daily

Salad greens and other green vegetables tend to be highly alkalizing to your body, thanks to their plentiful amounts of alkaline minerals. Having a large green salad at least once a day is an easy way to ensure that you achieve the 70:30 ratio. Use acid-forming salad dressings sparingly, and avoid bottled salad dressings altogether—they're usually full of sugar, preservatives, stabilizers, and other acid-forming junk. In addition to your large salad, add a handful of salad greens to a wrap or as an accompaniment to other meals.

Sprout Out Loud

Sprouted beans and seeds are another great way to increase the raw power of your diet. You may already be familiar with bean sprouts, found in most grocery stores. These are made from mung beans (small green beans) that have been soaked and sprouted. You can also try sprouting organic alfalfa, broccoli, chia, pumpkin, sunflower, or clover seeds and soybeans, chickpeas, lentils, and adzuki beans. Avoid kidney bean sprouts, as they are highly toxic.

It's easy to sprout beans and seeds. Simply cover a small amount with pure, alkaline water and let stand overnight, during which time they will absorb most of the water. Rinse and drain them, then cover them and let them stand until they sprout, rinsing and draining them at least twice a day. They will usually begin sprouting within one to three days. Once they reach the desired length (usually before they grow green leaves), you can store them in a glass jar or other airtight container in the fridge. Rinse and drain them again before eating.

Add sprouts to salads, wraps, and other foods to significantly increase their nutritional value. Most sprouts contain highly usable protein that requires little energy to digest. Sprouting beans and seeds also increases their vitamin content exponentially and makes them more alkalizing.

Don't worry if you don't have time to sprout beans and seeds yourself; they are readily available in most health food and grocery stores. It is not essential to grow your own at home.

Good Health in a Nutshell

While most nuts are acid-forming in your body and should be confined to the 30 percent wise acid portion of your diet, almonds are alkaline-forming and can be eaten freely. Eat them raw and unsalted for maximum healing potential. Snack on them throughout the day for an alkaline protein snack that will stabilize blood sugar levels, keep you feeling full, and ward off cravings.

Because all nuts contain enzyme inhibitors, it's best to soak almonds for an hour before eating them. They'll absorb the water and be easier to digest. Soaking also activates their plentiful nutrients, making them more available for your body to absorb.

I use ground almonds (also called almond flour) to make bread, muffins, cookies, and other baked goods. Almond milk, a delicious alkalizing substitute for dairy milk, is terrific as a drink in its own right or as a base for smoothies. It can also be used in baking or added to herbal teas. See page 145 for a basic almond milk recipe.

KICK ACID TIP #7

Snack on Almonds

Loaded with calcium, magnesium, and fiber, almonds help build strong bones, ensure healthy electrical signals between brain cells, and bind to toxins in the body before they can cause damage. Magnesium stabilizes brain waves and increases oxygenated blood flow to the brain, both of which are essential to brain health. Snacking on almonds also helps regulate blood sugar levels, which in turn helps to balance weight. Soak raw almonds in water, drain, and carry a bag with you to snack on throughout the day. They are truly alkalizing superfoods!

Cooking with the Alkalizing Grains

Buckwheat groats and quinoa have a rather intense flavor, so when you're baking bread, they are best used in small quantities, mixed with another grain, such as spelt. Quinoa can be used in place of rice or couscous in most dishes. Spelt has a naturally sweet taste and is delicious in breads and muffins. In chapter 8, you'll find recipes for dishes that include these healthy and tasty grains, as well as information on cooking them.

Adding Legumes to Your Diet

Because legumes are good sources of protein, they make a healthy substitute for meat, which is extremely acidic and does not contain any fiber. Legumes are very versatile, and there are many great ways to include them in your meals and snacks. You can add them to salads, soups, stews, and casseroles or purée them to use as the basis for dips and spreads (such as the Hummus recipe on page 152).

Type of Legume	Suggested Uses
Lentils	Curries, soups, stews, African, Moroccan, and Indian dishes
Lima beans	Casseroles, soups, salads
Navy beans	Baked beans, soups, stews
Black beans*	Soups, stews, rice and beans, Mexican dishes, Central and South American cuisines, Slow Cooker Black Bean Chili (page 164)
Chickpeas (garbanzo beans)*	Casseroles, minestrone soup, salads, Spanish- or African-style stews, Moroccan tagines, Indian curries, Hummus (page 152)
Kidney beans*	Stews, mixed bean salads, chili, Southwestern-style bean dishes

* To be eaten as part of your 30 percent wise acid choices.

See page 171 to learn how to cook dried legumes. Alternatively, use bottled legumes. If you can't find them, use organic canned legumes, free of EDTA, sodium, and preservatives. Rinse beans well before using.

Incorporating Soy Products

Soy flour is just what it sounds like—flour made from ground soybeans. Because it's one of the few alkaline flours, it's a good way to add protein, fiber, and phytochemicals to baked goods. It is best mixed with other, milder types of flour to avoid a beany taste.

Soy milk is made by grinding soybeans and mixing them with water to form a milk-like liquid. Store-bought soy milk tends to be slightly acid-forming due to the sweeteners and thickeners added to it. But it is significantly less acidic than dairy products and can be used as a replacement for cow's milk. It's a solid option for the 30 percent component of your diet. Homemade soy milk tends to be slightly alkaline, but making it can be a lot of work, so it's definitely not for everyone. If you're inclined to make your own, you might want to invest in an electric soy milk machine. I enjoy fresh soy milk, but it does have a slightly beany taste that takes some getting used to. For sweeter homemade soy milk, add stevia to suit your taste. Don't worry if you don't have a soy milk machine; it is not an essential component of the Kick Acid program.

Tofu is bean curd made from soybeans in a process similar to that used to make cheese. Because it has a bland, rather spongy texture, it absorbs the flavors of the foods it is cooked with. Forget what you've heard about or experienced with tofu. While I admit it can have an odd taste on its own, when combined with the right foods and prepared in the right way, it is delicious. Try my Fajitas recipe (page 162) if you don't believe me. Tofu is available in most health food stores and grocery stores in varying degrees of firmness, including extra-firm, firm, soft, and silken.

Here are some ideas on how to incorporate tofu and other soy products into your diet:

- Add extra-firm or firm tofu to Asian dishes and stir-fries. Freezing tofu and then thawing it before use gives it a firmer, chewier texture, comparable to chicken. It can then be marinated in a little Bragg's Aminos (a natural condiment that tastes like soy sauce) or lemon juice, or another marinade of your choice.
- Use crumbled firm or extra-firm tofu in place of ground beef in tacos, chili, or other recipes.
- Use silken tofu, with some lemon juice and a few seasonings, to replace sour cream.
- Whip silken tofu with berries or other fruit into a delicious pudding.
- Snack on a handful of soy nuts or edamame rather than on chips or crackers.
- Use soy milk in place of dairy milk in baked goods.

THE HEALING POWER OF WATER

Would you believe that drinking water is one of the most healing things you can do for your body? It's true—as long as it is pure, filtered, alkaline water.

Earlier, we talked about some of the environmental impacts of acid rain. Just as we can measure the pH of our saliva, urine, and blood, the pH scale can be used to determine whether the water we drink is alkaline or acidic. To review, water that measures less than 7 on the scale is acidic; water that's higher than 7 is alkaline. To support life, water needs to maintain an acid–base balance within a narrow range, much like our bodies. We are part of this planet's natural environment, which is dependent on alkaline water.

Drinking pure, alkaline water is an essential part of the Ultimate pH Solution and is critical to great health. Since most tap water is acidic and contains harmful toxins such as fluoride and chlorine, it's a good idea to invest in a water purification system. There are many water filtration systems that eliminate some of the harmful toxins or microbes, but a few systems also raise the pH of your water to increase its healing powers. These filters typically use a neutralizing agent such as calcium carbonate, calcite, or magnesium oxide to raise the pH. You may find it difficult to make sense of the many water filtration options available: there are carbon filters, distillation units, ultraviolet systems, and many others. Every company claims its products are the best. Don't let the confusion stop you from purchasing a water filtration system. The units designed to both purify and alkalize water tend to be the best option. To simplify things, I've provided information on various water filtration systems in Appendix B (page 179).

Don't assume that bottled water is necessarily a better option than tap water. Most bottled water is a questionable alternative. Many brands are derived from municipal sources, and some actually contain tap water from major cities. Also, many brands are acidic. Biochemist Robert O. Young conducted a test of more than 60 brands of bottled water, as well as tap water, to determine the pH of each. The chart below gives a sampling of his findings. As you can see, only the brands shaded in gray are alkaline. Several common brands are acidic.

Every cell in your body depends on adequate water to ensure proper functioning. As part of the Ultimate pH Solution, it is important to drink between 12 and 20 cups of alkaline water a day. Every person has individual water needs, but if you are smaller than average and are in excellent health, try to get at least 12 cups daily; if you have any health problems, are overweight, or are larger than average, drink 20 cups daily. As your health problems improve and you lose any excess weight, you can reduce your consumption to 12 cups. If you are feeling sick or sluggish, or have any other symptoms of ill health, increase your water intake to 20 cups daily.

You can raise both the alkalinity and the healing power of your water by adding pH drops to it. There are many different brands of pH drops available.

COMMON BRANDS OF BOTTLED WATER AND THEIR PH LEVELS[2]

Brand	pH Level
San Pellegrino (spring water)	4.49
Perrier	4.91
Pellegrino (sparkling water)	5.28
New York City municipal tap water	5.81
Aquafina	5.96
Volvic	7.07
Whistler Water	7.18
Dasani	7.2
Evian	7.53
Canadian Mountain	7.96
Vittel	7.98

Or try adding 16 drops of 2 percent sodium chlorite (available from many health practitioners and health food stores) to each quart of distilled or ionized water. Alternatively, add a teaspoon or two of pure baking soda to each quart of pure, alkaline water.[3] This mixture makes a great quick fix to restore balance, and most people find they adapt to the taste. And don't forget that adding fresh lemon juice to a glass of water is an excellent way to alkalize your body.

pH SOLUTION

Curtis Kicks Acid

When I met my husband, Curtis, I loved everything about him . . . except his diet. He had just turned 30 and was working full-time for the federal government, going to school, and actively participating in a number of sports. He told me he had always been a picky eater and a "meat and potatoes" guy. He ate a lot of fruit, but only apples and bananas. His vegetable repertoire consisted mostly of carrots and the occasional broccoli floret. His idea of a salad was iceberg lettuce. Pizza, chicken, fries, pasta, beef, dairy products, and bread figured heavily in his diet.

Our first trip to the grocery store together was traumatic for me. We divided to conquer our grocery lists, and when Curtis returned with the shopping cart, he had added "cherry chip" cake mix, fruit punch instead of the juice I'd asked him to pick up, and frozen crescent roll dough. I also noticed the jars of tomato sauce and the six-pack of cola. I wanted to spend my life with this man, but with this diet, I wondered how long he'd last. I added my organic produce, fresh herbs, brown rice pasta, tofu, and wild salmon to the cart and planned my strategy to introduce some healthier food into his diet.

Improving his diet was important to me because he had been eating like this for 30 years and was feeling the effects of his poor choices, whether he made the connection to his diet or not. He complained of fatigue and headaches on a daily basis. He could no longer finish runs or bike rides without feeling like his muscles had shut down. He suffered from insomnia, and when he did sleep, it was disrupted by leg cramps. Yet by all outward appearances, he was a healthy man.

We both laugh when we think back to one of our first experiences making dinner together in our first home. I had made a homemade tomato sauce with fresh organic tomatoes, sautéed onions, red peppers, olive oil, and fresh basil. Curtis opened his jar of spaghetti sauce and put it into a separate pot on the stove. He cooked his white pasta and I ate brown rice pasta. He commented on how good my dinner smelled, yet showed no interest in trying my healthier meal. I knew at that moment that getting him to eat a healthier diet was going to take some effort and some time. Being a fairly patient woman (or at least, I'd like to think so), I was willing to slowly introduce healthier options into his life.

Curtis is now a huge fan of my homemade tomato sauce and spelt pasta. He regularly comments on how much better the healthier options taste. He has substantially more energy than he did a decade ago, rarely experiences a headache, and only occasionally suffers from insomnia. I chuckle when I over-hear him giving his co-workers and colleagues advice about eating healthier and telling them how important it is to kick acid.

CHAPTER 6

Choosing the Best Alkaline-Friendly Supplements

"Make the most of yourself, for that is all there is of you."

—RALPH WALDO EMERSON

Everybody needs a little help sometimes. There is no shame in using some extra assistance to improve a situation—and using nutritional supplements is no different. Supplementing your diet with vitamin, mineral, and herbal products can provide that much-needed boost your body requires to combat the symptoms and effects of acidity. In a perfect world, where we all ate organic vegetables and fruit grown in fertile, nutrient-rich soil fed by pure, alkaline mountain water, breathed fresh, oxygen-rich air, and got plenty of exercise, perhaps we wouldn't need nutritional or herbal supplements. But we know that's not the case. While you should get most of your nutrition from alkaline foods or wise acid choices, it is valuable to supplement your diet to prevent any nutritional deficiencies or to give your diet a boost. On the flip side, supplements are never replacements for a healthy diet. They work best when they *supplement* a healthy diet.

Not all supplements are created equal. That multivitamin at the grocery or big-box store is not the same as the professional-grade multivitamin your natural medicine doctor recommends. The doses, and even the ingredients, may be different. You may be shocked to learn that many of your favorite supplements are acidic. They can contain preservatives, alcohol, and sugar or other sweeteners, all of which can create harmful acidity in your body. Some supplements contain binders or fillers, or even heavy metals such as lead (a common problem in many calcium supplements). In addition, the manufacturing processes used by many nutritional supplement companies cause these pills to become acidic. This can happen through contamination when the supplement is being produced. Enzyme supplements, for example, may be grown on beds of yeast, which results in unwanted yeast or its spores in your enzymes. Pure, uncontaminated sources of raw materials for supplements are not always used, and many companies simply do not implement or ensure safe, healthy manufacturing processes.

It is important not only to choose high-quality nutritional supplements, but also to ensure that you take the right ones. To the vast majority of the population, supplements are harmless in recommended doses. However, if you're on medication or under medical care for a serious health condition, it's important to consult your physician before introducing supplements into your diet and health regime. Herbal supplements, in particular, get a bad rap for "interfering" with pharmaceutical drugs. While herbs are a natural food with medicinal qualities—and are frequently the original source from which drugs are "discovered"—it is the herbal product rather than the drug (and its long list of side effects) that gets blamed for complications. I am always shocked when people are more concerned about herbs that have been used for thousands of years than about relatively recent synthetic pharmaceutical drugs with a lengthy list of side effects. Nevertheless, do consult a qualified health professional if you have any concerns.

It is not necessary to take all of the supplements suggested in this chapter. But if you were going to pick only one item, I would suggest green food supplements, such as the green powders that are added to juice or smoothies to make green drinks. Other green food supplements come in the form of tablets or capsules, as is often the case with chlorella (a type of alga) and spirulina (also a type of alga). Green food supplements pack a huge nutritional punch and are very alkalizing at the same time. They should be a part of everyone's daily regime.

BUYER BEWARE

Supplements are like any other product: if you do your homework, you'll find the best one. And you usually get what you pay for. It's your right to know how a supplement manufacturer makes its product, what goes into it, where the ingredients come from, and whether the process has safeguards against contamination. Ask these questions at your local health food store or pharmacy. Or call the manufacturer. If you don't get a satisfactory response, take your business elsewhere. The manufacturer should be able to show third-party laboratory testing confirming that the ingredient amounts listed on the label are present in the supplement and that no contaminated sources of nutrients were used in the raw materials for the supplements.

WATER-ALKALIZING SUPPLEMENTS

Sometimes, improving your alkaline state can be as simple as adding highly alkaline compounds to your drinking water. You can purchase ready-made "pH drops" from a reputable health store. These drops may contain a 2 percent solution of chlorine dioxide or hydrogen peroxide, which releases oxygen into the body, helping you to improve your alkalinity or remain alkaline.

In addition to liquid drops, there are a number of alkaline powders on the market. These products are typically mineral salts containing potassium, magnesium, calcium, manganese, and even iron. Again, it is important to read the labels or contact the company directly to find out all of the ingredients, including sugars and other additives.

Other products work to improve oxygen uptake at the cellular level. Cellfood is a liquid formula containing 78 minerals, 34 enzymes, and 17 amino acids. It uses a proprietary technological process to deliver these plant-based nutrients as well as bioavailable oxygen ("bioavailable" means it can be used effectively by your body). It has a negative charge, much like blood and lymph, which leads to rapid absorption of the nutrients. It also helps to neutralize free radicals and prevent further free-radical damage at the cellular level, and it may improve your ability to eliminate toxins. Simply add eight drops of Cellfood to a glass of pure water three times daily. It is available in most health food stores. See page 182 for more information.

GREEN DRINKS

Drinking something that's green might not sound great. But green drinks are packed with vital nutrition and help to restore balance to your body quickly. Also, the chlorophyll (the natural part of the plant that makes it green) in green drinks has a sweet taste, making them very palatable. Chlorophyll is highly alkaline and is vital for photosynthesis. (Remember your high-school biology? That's how plants obtain energy from light.) It is similar in structure to our red blood cells, except it contains a magnesium atom (or ion) at its center, while red blood cells contain iron as their central atom. The similarity enables your body to use chlorophyll to create new and healthy blood cells, thereby detoxifying your blood of harmful acidic toxins.

Chlorophyll research has focused on its positive effects on cancers and its anti-mutagenic properties (it helps to protect your body's genetic material from damage). You might not be aware that your genetic material—your

DNA—can be damaged, leaving you vulnerable to various health problems. Chlorophyll has been shown to have a protective effect on DNA.[1]

Obviously, the most natural source of chlorophyll is a diet rich in green vegetables, but with our busy lives we're not always able to get enough of these. I recommend using green powder to boost your chlorophyll intake, alongside a diet with plenty of green vegetables. Green powder or liquid chlorophyll is a great addition to a healthy diet, but is not a replacement for eating your green salads and vegetables.

There are many different types of green powders. They are usually comprised of barley greens, wheatgrass, alfalfa, spirulina, blue-green algae, or chlorella and are found in powdered form in your local health food store. Be sure to choose one that is free of sweeteners (artificial or otherwise), artificial colors or flavors, and other acidic ingredients. It's important to read the ingredient list and choose a high-quality product.

To make a green drink, add a teaspoon or two of green powder to 4 cups of water. This cocktail is best taken on an empty stomach, or at least a couple of hours after a meal. To prevent the powder from clumping, use a blender or hand mixer. Individual-size blenders work well, and you can usually drink straight from the mixing cup, making it easy to whip up a green drink and take it on the road for days when you're in a hurry. In addition to chlorophyll, green drinks are chock-full of vitamins, minerals, and other beneficial nutrients and phytochemicals. I encourage you to drink between one and four daily to restore naturally alkaline pH levels to your body. If you're suffering from health problems or are overweight, strive for four green drinks a day.

KICK ACID TIP #8

Go for the Green

Green drinks are a fast and simple way to restore your body's pH balance. Drinking them is a good habit on a daily basis, and is even more important on days when you've fallen off the wagon and eaten a more acidic diet. Add a scoop of unsweetened green powder to 4 cups of water and drink on an empty stomach.

CHLORELLA

Chlorella is another beneficial supplement for raising pH levels. These amazing single-cell algae contain chlorophyll, amino acids, vitamin D, and enzymes.

Chlorella improves blood oxygenation, digestion, and waste elimination. In addition, research has shown that it binds to and escorts toxins and heavy metals such as mercury (the dangerous metal used in many old dental amalgams) out of the body.[2] Regardless of whether you're drinking green drinks, I recommend chlorella. Even the healthiest people will benefit from one of nature's richest superfoods, but it's particularly beneficial for those who suspect mercury toxicity or another type of environmental toxin exposure.

Chlorella typically comes in small green pills that you can chew or swallow whole, as you wish. Not everyone likes the taste, but many people find that chewing the tablets is a great way to ensure digestion and absorption of the nutrients, as well as to alkalize the mouth and beat bad breath. Products vary, so follow the directions on the label of the product you choose.

DIGESTIVE ENZYMES

Enzymes are essential to great health and are required by virtually every process in your body. Your body makes many different types of enzymes, such as metabolic enzymes that help you regulate your body and digestive enzymes that, as the name implies, help you digest your food. We can also obtain enzymes by eating raw fruits and vegetables, which contain enzymes that help start digestion in our mouths when we eat them. Keep in mind that I said "raw." Cooking kills enzymes.

An acid diet uses up our natural and finite enzyme supply at an alarming rate. When we are excessively acidic from eating foods such as cooked meat or white-flour breads, our digestion becomes less effective. Our body must manufacture more enzymes to deal with poorly digested food, not simply in the stomach but along the entire gastrointestinal tract. As we waste enzymes dealing with this food, our digestive organs and our pancreas, which produces enzymes, are strained. Poorly digested food can lead to a host of problems, including allergies and increased bacterial growth in the intestines, which further acidifies the body and depletes or destroys enzymes. If you see undigested food in your stool, you may not be chewing well enough to break down your food, your internal enzymes may be struggling with your food choices, or you may have depleted your enzyme supplies from an excessively acidic diet over time.

A diet that contains a large amount of raw vegetables—and, to a lesser extent, fruit—will help boost the body's enzyme supply. I recommend that you also take a supplement that contains a full spectrum of digestive enzymes, including lipase, protease, amylase, maltase, oxidase, peroxidase, invertase, phosphatase, and cellulose, to help break down a variety of foods in your diet. These supplements usually come in capsules or tablets. Take one or two at every meal.

BROMELAIN

Bromelain is a combination of enzymes found in pineapple. While the highest concentrations are found in the inedible stem, it is extracted and sold as a digestive enzyme in tablet or capsule form. Studies have shown that bromelain has powerful anti-inflammatory properties and may be useful in numerous autoimmune disorders, such as lupus, fibromyalgia, arthritis, and chronic fatigue syndrome.[3] In Germany, bromelain is approved for the treatment of sinus and nasal swelling associated with ear, nose, and throat surgery or trauma. When taken internally, bromelain enzymes perform a housekeeping function by removing waste material such as dead bacteria and fungus and supporting the growth of healthy flora in the intestine. If you are suffering from pain, swelling, or inflammation, I recommend taking bromelain on an empty stomach in addition to a digestive enzyme supplement with meals.

ESSENTIAL FATTY ACIDS

We have already learned that most of us are getting too much of the wrong kinds of fat and not enough of the healthy fats. Even when our diet provides healthy fats, it is usually in the wrong ratio of omega-6s to omega-3s, making us vulnerable to acid waste from inflammation in our bodies. That's where a good-quality essential fatty acid (EFA) supplement comes in handy. Remember, these are fats we can get only through our diet—our body needs them but does not make them. EFAs support our cardiovascular, immune, nervous, and reproductive systems. They are essential at the cellular level to build and repair cell membranes and to expel harmful waste products. They help break up and remove the dangerous saturated fatty acids that clog our blood.

EFA supplements can come as gel capsules or in liquid form. Even the experts don't agree on the optimum ratio of omega-6 fatty acids to omega-3s, but look for a ratio between 4:1 and 1:1, and always check for freshness. The supplements should be refrigerated, and the omega-3s last for only about six months, so if they look like they've been collecting dust on the shelves of your health food store, you might be better off with another product. Liquid supplements should not smell rancid or fishy, even if they are from a fish source.

Alternatively, you can start consuming flax, hemp, borage, or walnut oil. Try to get at least a tablespoon or two daily.

MULTIVITAMINS

Vitamins are often called "essential micronutrients" because they are required continuously by the body in relatively small amounts. Because the body does not store vitamins, we have to consume them regularly. Different vitamins are found in different food sources, and a well-rounded diet is necessary to obtain all the vitamins required for health. The typical North American diet does not provide us with enough nutrients. Fortunately, most vitamins can be obtained in alkaline-forming, neutral, or low acid-forming vegetables and fruits. Others, such as vitamin B_{12} (discussed below), are found primarily in highly acidic meat and dairy products (sprouts are a good vegetarian source of B_{12}).

I recommend a high-quality multivitamin with a wide variety of trace minerals, devoid of sweeteners, fillers, colors, preservatives, wheat, corn, and other potential allergens and acidic ingredients. Keep in mind that the form of a specific nutrient can make a difference to its ability to be digested and absorbed by your body. Consider potassium, for example. Recent research conducted at the University of Basel in Switzerland demonstrated that 161 postmenopausal women gained an increase in bone mineral density after taking a potassium citrate supplement for a year. A second group of women experienced no gain while taking potassium chloride for the same amount of time. The researchers concluded that the alkaline form of potassium, potassium citrate, benefits the bones and can actually increase bone mass.[4] Many experts recommend the citrate form of minerals because it appears to be better absorbed by the body.

KICK ACID TIP #9

Choose the Alkaline Form of Vitamin C

Vitamin C is integral to many body functions and helps the immune system stay strong and the stress glands keep up with their daily load. But the form of vitamin C found in most supplements is ascorbic acid. While ascorbic acid has many health benefits, it adds more acidity to an already acidic body. Instead, choose calcium ascorbate, the alkaline form of vitamin C. You'll reap all the benefits of vitamin C without the acidity.

B COMPLEX VITAMINS

Your brain, your heart, and even your mood depend on adequate amounts of B complex vitamins. While you may be getting some B vitamins in a multi-vitamin, an additional B complex supplement may be a good idea. Thousands of research studies show the health benefits of supplementing your diet with B vitamins. We need to obtain adequate amounts of all the B vitamins or risk deficiencies. Unfortunately, our highly acidic diets are mostly devoid of B complex vitamins, and our high-stress lifestyles further deplete them, as do alcohol, cigarettes, and prescription or over-the-counter medications.

In chapter 3, we briefly discussed the link between elevated homocysteine levels, increased acidity, and, ultimately, cardiovascular problems. While additional studies are required, promising scientific evidence suggests that folate (also known as vitamin B_9), vitamin B_6, and vitamin B_{12} are effective at lowering homocysteine levels and may ultimately play a role in reducing vascular disease. In addition, research has revealed an inverse relationship between folate and the occurrence of colorectal cancer.[5] (In other words, the more deficient in folate you are, the greater your risk of colorectal cancer.)

HERBS AND SPICES

Herbs and spices have been used for thousands of years, probably as long as humans have roamed the earth. The vast majority of herbs and spices are alkalizing to the body, and they make a great addition to your diet and medicine cabinet.

Fresh organic herbs not only help alkalize your body, they make your recipes taste better. Experiment with herbs and spices. When you add fresh garlic, ginger, basil, cilantro, oregano, or rosemary to that vegetable, grain, or bean dish you are preparing, you'll be amazed at how good your food can taste—without table salt and black pepper. Over time, you may begin to wonder how you cooked without fresh herbs. I grow herbs in my garden and on my windowsill during the winter months so they are ready whenever I need them. When I'm running low, I add fresh organic herbs to my grocery cart.

In addition to using herbs and spices in your cooking, you can benefit from their many healing properties by drinking herbal teas. Try them instead of coffee or black tea, both of which are acid-forming in your body. There are many great options, from peppermint tea to blends formulated for medicinal purposes, such as detoxification or combating insomnia or PMS. Check out the selection of herbal teas in your local health food store. If you want a sweetener, add two to three drops of stevia for all the sweetness and none of the acidity of sugar or artificial sweeteners.

There are thousands of different herbs, each with its own medicinal properties. Oregano is a potent antiviral, antibacterial, and antifungal agent. Cilantro mobilizes mercury out of body tissues so it can be eliminated. Depending on your specific health needs and tastes, you may wish to supplement some of them. Garlic, for example, has many heart-protecting benefits, so if you can't stand the taste, look for a high-quality odorless garlic supplement.

COMMON USES FOR FRESH HERBS

Experiment with these readily available fresh herbs in your cooking:

- **Basil:** Pasta, vegetables, tomato sauce, salad dressings, sauces, stews
- **Bay leaves:** Sauces, soups, stews
- **Chives:** Soups, salads, stews, salad dressings
- **Dill:** Salads, soups, stews, salad dressings
- **Lemon balm:** Tea, salads
- **Marjoram:** Soups, vegetables
- **Mint:** Tea, salads, fruit desserts
- **Oregano:** Beans, pasta sauces, soups, stews
- **Parsley:** Soups, salads, casseroles, vegetables, juices
- **Rosemary:** Bread, vegetables, soups, stews
- **Sage:** Salads, casseroles, soups, stews
- **Thyme:** Soups, salads, stews, bread

SPECIAL ALKALINE SUPPLEMENTS

There is now enough valid scientific research supporting the role of acidity in poor health that companies are introducing specific alkaline formulas to supplement our food choices and restore pH balance in our bodies. I don't want to sound like a broken record, but it really is a case of "buyer beware." There are good products and bad products, and it can be difficult to know the difference unless you research particular brands. If I see amazing claims that are not backed by credible and verifiable data and research, I am skeptical.

Some of the best products are professional-grade formulas that are sold only to health professionals. If you are suffering from severe health problems, it is wise to work with a skilled professional anyway; he or she can guide you in your supplement selection.

While an alkaline diet is one of the best ways to kick acid in your body, it is also important to reduce stress—or at least improve your ability to relax during stressful times. Meditation and breathing exercises are great ways to reduce acid–forming stress hormones and increase oxygen, which helps alkalize your blood. In the next chapter, you'll learn about important lifestyle changes or additions that will help you kick acid for life.

pH Solution

Ray Loses Weight the Alkaline Way

Ray loved to eat and had always had problems with his weight. While he'd tried dieting, he had repeatedly failed because he was "always hungry, even on high-protein diets." His diet included plentiful amounts of steak, bacon, chicken, eggs, and cheese. He had read that these foods could help him lose weight, even without concern for portion size or caloric intake. At first, he loved eating so much meat, but after a while he grew tired of it. He came to me because he had started to suffer from headaches, constipation, and achy joints—common signs of excess protein and acidity. He was now at the point of vowing never to diet again.

I agreed that diets don't work, but thought Ray might reach his optimal weight by getting his acid under control. I suggested that balancing his pH would make his body healthier and prevent illness (his father had died of colon cancer). I pointed out that weight often drops off when the pH is balanced, and the alkaline-producing foods create a healthier dietary lifestyle.

Ray was addicted to morning muffins and evening ice cream, but he agreed to try the new program. Within three months, he had lost nearly 15 pounds more easily than he'd anticipated. He found that he actually enjoyed alkaline-boosting foods. His favorites were Carrot Apple Ginger Juice (page 142) and Red Pepper–Butternut Squash Quesadillas (page 163), and he loved snacking on frozen blueberries as a treat instead of ice cream. He allowed himself a weekly muffin, but noticed that he felt better on the days he skipped it. And he told me, "I never feel hungry eating this way." Now a disciple of his new dietary lifestyle, he was spreading the gospel of its positive results. Ray continued on the program and, six months later, found to his amazement that he'd lost 50 pounds. As a pleasant side effect, his headaches, constipation, and achy joints were gone.

Ray has kept the weight off for the past six years. He occasionally allows himself some of his favorite foods, such as steak and muffins, but he then returns to his "dietary preferences," as he calls them. His mother and sister have now joined his regimen to prevent health problems and lose weight. Everyone in Ray's family is much happier, thanks to his excellent example of commitment to a program that is not only improving his appearance but saving his life!

CHAPTER 7

The Kick Acid Lifestyle

"The secret of health for both mind and body is not to mourn for the past, worry about the future, or anticipate troubles, but to live in the present moment wisely and earnestly."

—HINDU PRINCE GAUTAMA SIDDHARTHA, FOUNDER OF BUDDHISM

It's not what you do for a day or a month that ensures health; it's what you do for a lifetime. It's easy to maintain your pH balance throughout your life by striving for balance each day. Aside from healthy dietary choices, there are many lifestyle choices you can make to help decrease acidity. In this chapter, you'll learn alkalizing options that help nature restore or maintain optimum health, including exercise (the right kind, and in the right amount), natural therapies, and even bathing. That's right—there's a luxurious bath option for when you want to alkalize your body while relaxing. You'll also learn ways to incorporate the dietary suggestions into your life. You can even try a one-week sample meal plan to give your body a jump-start on health, energy, and vitality.

Don't worry if you don't have the budget for a far infrared sauna (page 128) or can't find the oils to give yourself a lymphatic massage (page 125). With the exception of exercise and deep breathing, which everyone should be doing, the lifestyle suggestions in this chapter are helpful additions to the Kick Acid program but are not essential. Their benefits are many and great, but there's no need to stress if you can't incorporate all of these ideas into your life. Remember, stress causes the release of acidifying hormones.

Conversely, don't rely on these therapies alone to counter acidity in your body. The best way to balance your biochemistry is to eat and drink more alkaline foods and make wise acid choices. Try to exercise at least three to five times a week, breathe deeply whenever you can, enjoy these wonderful therapies as your time and budget permit, and you'll be well on your way to kicking acid.

THE ALKALIZING POWER OF EXERCISE

We've discussed how acidity affects the kidneys and what we can do to ensure better kidney health. We've touched on the role of the liver and how acidity affects it. In this section, I want to explain how the lungs, the lymphatic system, and the skin help improve our pH balance when we exercise.

Before you set the book down, muttering, "I'm not joining the gym or starting to jog," keep reading. I am not suggesting this at all. I don't have a gym membership, and I don't jog. Neither activity interests me. However, I know that I have to work my muscles and joints to keep them in top shape, elevate my heart rate and breathing slightly to oxygenate my blood, and move my body to get my lymph fluid flowing. There are some simple, low-cost ways to achieve these results: take a brisk walk; join a yoga class; try tai chi; dust off your bike and hit the streets; head for the basketball or tennis court. Whatever your game, it's time to get back in it.

Most of us already know that exercise offers many benefits: it increases energy, reduces stress, burns fat, speeds up metabolism, builds bone mass, increases oxygen to the tissues and organs, builds muscle, improves posture, improves lung capacity and strength, enhances flexibility, strengthens joints, balances the spine and hips, increases bodily awareness, balances the brain, calms the mind, increases relaxation, improves self-confidence, and assists with weight loss or gain (as needed).

But exercise, done properly, also helps counter acidity in our bodies. It gives acid wastes another way out of the body—through sweat. If you break a sweat while exercising, you're helping to lessen your body's acid load. With more than 3,500 pores per square inch of skin, you've got a great way to remove both liquid and gaseous acids from your body, while reaping the many other benefits mentioned above.

But it's important to avoid overexercising, which can increase lactic acid formation and contribute to an acidic state in your body. What's too much? Everyone is different—pay attention to your body's signals. If you're starting to feel exhausted, cramping, or experiencing any pain, it's best to stop. Strive to get at least 30 minutes of brisk activity three to five times a week. Your heart should be beating faster than usual, which means it is circulating acid wastes to your detox organs. You'll feel your breathing get deeper as well, which helps oxygenate and alkalize your blood.

Note: if you are overweight or suffering any serious health conditions, you should consult your physician before starting an exercise program. Also, if it's been a while since you've exercised, it's advisable to start slowly and gradually build up.

Include exercise as part of the Ultimate pH Solution lifestyle. It's best done on a regular basis. Try to commit to some form of exercise between three and five times weekly. Mix up the type of exercise you do, so you'll stay interested. But don't forget that whenever you're off track in the acidity department, you can hit the treadmill, pace the streets, or crash the courts. Throw in an extra exercise session when you need to raise your pH to a healthier, slightly alkaline reading. And remember that, for maximum acid-balancing effects, you need to exercise in a way that helps you break a sweat.

Here are some great ways to get your heart rate up, work up a sweat, and get your lymph fluid moving, without creating exercise-induced acid buildup in your body.

Walk This Way

Walking is something most of us can do and need to do in the course of day-to-day living. It is, in my opinion, the safest and most effective exercise for the majority of the population. Biomechanically, the human body was designed to walk, and walking causes far less joint impact than running or jumping. It is "scalable," meaning you can change the pace and the distance as required. You can do it by yourself or with your spouse, partner, friends, kids, co-workers, or parents. It can be meditative or social. Walking is also low-cost: all you need is a good pair of shoes and proper clothing for the weather conditions. You can walk in the city, the forest, or the country, and you can walk in every season. While people often have to plan a workout or book a tennis court, walking is easily integrated into your day. Walk to the corner store or library. Walk up and down the stairs at the office. Turn off the television and walk and talk with your sweetheart.

Walking helps elevate our breathing rate and oxygenate our blood. When we breathe more deeply, we expel more carbon dioxide, which decreases acidity in our body. Increased oxygen in our blood helps to feed a healthy cellular environment and contributes to a more alkaline state. Walking exercises our muscles in a way that ensures they have enough oxygen and fuel to function without damage. It will also get your lymph fluid moving and may help you work up a sweat. Remember, the skin is our largest detoxification organ, and perspiration not only helps us keep cool, it helps us eliminate toxins through our skin surface.

If you cannot walk due to injury or disability, don't worry. I've included some great exercise options for everyone. Keep reading to find the best exercise for you.

Bounce Your Way to Better Health

How would you like to strengthen your muscles and bones, get your lymphatic system pumping, improve your circulation, and burn calories in the comfort of your own living room? What if I said you could be watching television at the same time? Too good to be true? No, it's not. It's called rebounding, and it is one of the best exercises for eliminating acid from your body.

Rebounders are miniature trampolines. They are usually round, are quick to assemble, and are easy to store. Rebounders are inexpensive and can be found in the sports section of many department stores, as well as at specialty exercise equipment outlets. Keep in mind that you usually get what you pay for, so be sure to buy a model that's well constructed and not so stiff that the impact jars your joints. You also don't want it to fall apart while you're bouncing on it!

The non-jarring nature of rebounding is one of its benefits. It does not place additional stress on joints, as jogging, tennis, or basketball does. The rebounding motion actually serves as a pumping action to get your lymphatic system moving, thereby increasing its ability to transport accumulated toxins and acidity out of your body. This simple activity has been shown to increase the flow of lymph fluid to up to 14 times its normal speed. Because it is aerobic, it also exercises the heart and makes it stronger. A strong heart pumps blood more efficiently. Rebounding provides a great muscle workout, improving tone, strength, and coordination. I find the gentle bouncing motion meditative and relaxing, so it's a great activity when you're feeling stressed. And the best part is, you'll feel like a kid again.

As with any new form of exercise, it's important to be conservative and cautious. If you have serious health problems and would like to begin rebounding, consult your physician first. You can also buy stabilizing bars for your rebounder to assist with balance.

Rebounders are great for the entire family, and 15 or 20 minutes a day can produce amazing health benefits. Start with 10 minutes a day for the first week. Then increase to 15 to 20 minutes daily. Rebounding can even be done in front of the television if you simply can't pull yourself away.

KICK ACID TIP #10

Dry-Brush Your Skin to Get Your Lymph Moving

Here's a simple way to stimulate your lymphatic system: get a natural-bristle brush meant for dry skin brushing from your local health food store. Before your morning shower, brush your dry skin in circular motions. Start at your feet and work up all sides of your legs. Then work in circles up your abdomen toward your heart. Continue brushing in circles up all sides of your arms. By doing this, you're stimulating your blood and lymph fluid to remove acidic wastes. Remember, always brush toward your heart: that's the way the lymphatic system naturally flows. This simple exercise takes only a minute or two but offers great health rewards.

Take Up a Mellow Martial Art

I'm not talking about kung fu and karate here, although these forms of exercise certainly have merit. But there are a couple of far less rigorous martial arts known as tai chi and qigong (pronounced "chi gung"). These ancient practices were used by warriors and sages alike to raise their level of consciousness, improve energy flow through the body, and even heal disease. Whether you believe these claims or not, both tai chi and qigong can reduce stress, improve breathing, increase energy, and provide a general sense of well-being, thereby reducing the amount of acidic stress hormones, such as cortisol, created in our bodies and increasing our oxygen uptake, which helps us right down to the cellular level. Remember: more oxygen = less acidity.

These martial arts are made up of a series of movements, usually coordinated with breathing. Watching an experienced tai chi practitioner is like watching a beautiful choreographed dance. The U.S. National Institutes of Health's National Center for Complementary and Alternative Medicine (NCCAM) is funding research on tai chi in a number of areas, including its effects on the immune system; its role in stress reduction and ability to cope in women diagnosed with breast cancer; and its ability to help alleviate osteoarthritis of the knee and improve physical function and immunity in those with rheumatoid arthritis.[1]

Qigong is usually more static than tai chi, but research has linked considerable physical and emotional health benefits to its practice. Qigong can be practiced while sitting or lying down, so it is also an excellent choice for people who have difficulty standing or walking.

Tai chi and qigong are offered in classes across North America, or you can pick up a book or video to learn how to do them. Most sessions are well under an hour, and you can adjust them to fit your time constraints. A few minutes a day is better than nothing.

KICK ACID TIP #11

Try Xiu Lian for Body and Soul

Dr. Zhi Gang Sha describes a technique for cleansing and healing in his book *Power Healing*. The practice of xiu lian (pronounced "shoo lee-en"), a form of qigong, has existed in Chinese culture for the past 5,000 years. According to Dr. Sha, "Xiu means to purify your heart, mind, and soul. It means having love, care, compassion, sincerity, honesty, generosity, integrity, unselfishness, and discipline. It also means accumulating virtue and giving service to people and society. Lian means to practice all of these things in your daily life, in your actions, behaviours, and thoughts."[2]

He explains how to perform this simple yet powerful technique: "Sit comfortably with your back straight, but not leaning against anything. Keep both feet on the floor. Relax. Place your hands in front of your chest. Gently touch the heels of your hands together, gently touch your thumbs together, and gently touch your little fingers together. Open your hands and fingers as though you were holding a beautiful lotus flower. Relax and maintain the position for a few minutes—the longer the better—while your mind is in a peaceful, pleasant, or meditative state."[3]

Stretch Your Body and Mind with Yoga

Most forms of yoga offer wonderful low-impact exercise, muscle toning, deep breathing, and flexibility training that make it suitable for just about anyone. Combined with its stress-reducing power, it is not surprising that this ancient art has gained widespread popularity around the world.

While it often does not translate well into our hectic North American lives, yoga (like the martial arts above) is an aspect of a broader lifestyle that promotes balance, harmony, and moderation, as well as care of our bodies, minds, and spirits. Will you be less likely to scream at your spouse after a yoga session? I have no proof, but my instincts say yes! Yoga, like walking, tai chi, and qigong, has a healing effect on your emotions and moods as well as on your body.

As with tai chi and qigong, you can look for a yoga class in your area (some are even held outside!), or pick up a video so you can learn how to do it at home.

NATURAL THERAPIES THAT REDUCE STRESS AND KICK ACID

Research shows that deep-breathing exercises, meditation, calming music, massage therapy, acupuncture, reflexology, shiatsu, therapeutic touch, and feeling and expressing gratitude can shift the balance between the "tending and befriending" hormone oxytocin and the "stressed out," acidifying hormone cortisol. When this happens, your body tends not only toward pH balance but toward balanced moods as well.

Deep Breathing

One of the common denominators in eliminating acid is deep breathing. This can be accomplished even when you are not exercising. Deep breathing should be your goal 24/7. When you hold your breath or take shallow breaths, you are robbing your body of much-needed oxygen. In addition, you are accumulating carbon dioxide, which is acidic and needs to be expelled from the body through exhalation. If it builds up in the blood, it reacts with water to form carbonic acid, which causes a drop in the blood's pH.

We are a society of chronic shallow breathers, and we simply need to be more conscious of our breathing. In many cultures, breath is synonymous with spirit. Breath provides the oxygen our bodies require for survival: we cannot live long without it. Shallow breathing affects our energy and mood and lessens the ability of our cells to eliminate acid wastes. Retrain your breathing by taking at least a few minutes daily to try this deep-breathing exercise:

1. Place one hand on your chest and the other on your abdomen. Breathe deeply into your abdomen through your nose—if you are doing it right and breathing into your diaphragm and the lower part of your lungs, the hand on your abdomen should rise higher than the one on your chest. As you inhale, count slowly to four.
2. Hold your breath, again counting slowly to four.
3. Exhale slowly through your nose to a count of four, gently contracting your abdominal muscles to eliminate all air from your lungs.
4. Repeat this cycle at least four times, or more if you can make the time.

Research shows that breathing deeply for even 30 seconds has a substantial effect on acidic stress hormones and, when practiced over time, can have a profound healing effect on mood, energy levels, and cardiovascular and respiratory health. Research collected for the National Center for Health Statistics' 2002 National Health Interview Survey illustrated that deep breathing was the fourth most common complementary and alternative medicine therapy used by respondents, with almost 12 percent having done it in the preceding 12 months.[4]

KICK ACID TIP #12

Release the Stress

The next time you're feeling overwhelmed by work, family, or another type of stress, ask yourself, "Will this matter at the end of my life?" Sometimes, putting things into perspective goes a long way toward reducing stress. Then practice the deep-breathing exercise suggested above. If you find that you're going over and over the same stressful thoughts in your mind, write them out or ask your partner or a close friend if you can talk them out. Be sure to reciprocate for him or her.

Meditation

As our lives become more fast-paced and frantic, stress hormones can wreak havoc on our systems. These chemicals—cortisol, adrenaline, and others—perform an important function: they are designed to help us respond to danger by either running away or fighting to defend ourselves. This stress response was intended to kick in only on occasion, to save us from a wild animal or in some other emergency. But in modern society, many of us are in a constant state of "fight or flight" as we deal with stressful jobs, relationships, financial problems, and health concerns. Stress hormones that were intended to be in our systems in large amounts on very rare occasions are now in our systems in large amounts very frequently.

Stress can cause people to resort to cigarettes, drugs, alcohol, or sweets as they seek stimulants or depressants to numb the pain of it. We have already learned about the acidifying effects of these poor choices. The adrenal glands are taxed, and the high cortisol levels they release can stimulate the appetite. But consumption of sweets simply prompts greater production of cortisol.

Meditation can be a useful tool to reduce stress and the havoc it causes in our minds and bodies. Rooted in age-old religious and spiritual traditions, meditation has become a widespread practice for coping, relaxing, and promoting overall wellness. It can be conducted as a stand-alone technique or integrated into practices such as yoga, tai chi, deep-breathing exercises, or qigong.[5]

While Western scientific study of meditation is limited and typically focuses on the mental and emotional benefits of relaxation, pain management, and stress reduction, meditation is integrally linked to the function of the autonomic nervous system, which regulates many organs and muscles in our bodies. It plays a role in how our heart beats, how we breathe and sweat, and how effectively our digestive system works.

Massage Therapy

Gone are the days when people would snicker about a friend getting a massage. Even mainstream media are reporting on the benefits of massage as medicine. In a February 2007 article from *Health* magazine, Mehmet C. Oz, famous surgeon and director of the Cardiovascular Institute at New York Presbyterian Hospital, was quoted as saying, "All of our surgery patients are offered the treatment—I call it 'service with a smile'—and it's a mandatory weekly prescription I give myself."[6]

While massage can assist with numerous health concerns, its effectiveness in stress reduction helps decrease the acid load in our body. Massage reduces the production of cortisol and other acid-forming stress hormones. When excess stress hormones are coursing through your body, your immune system has no chance to recover. It's not surprising that many of the symptoms and conditions associated with a highly acidic diet are the same as those associated with chronic stress: decreased bone density, decreased muscle tissue, blood sugar fluctuations, suppressed immune system, obesity, and many others.

Don't let stress get to you. Book a massage with a qualified therapist, or pick up a book or video and practice massage techniques with your partner.

KICK ACID TIP #13

Massage Stress Away

If you're feeling tense (or even if you're not), turn off the television, grab your partner or a willing friend, and give each other back massages. You'll both feel less stressed, and less stress means fewer acidic stress hormones coursing through your blood. Don't worry if you don't know what to do; just ask your partner what feels good and what doesn't. As an added bonus, exchanging massages incorporates give and take into a relationship and helps bring people together emotionally, not just physically.

Lymph Drainage

Because the lymphatic system plays a critical role in our health by ridding the body of toxins, we need it to be in great working order. The Standard American Diet is one of the biggest barriers to this goal. It clogs the body with acid-forming food, additives, chemicals, and other toxic substances. When this diet is combined with a sedentary lifestyle, our lymphatic system can use some help (remember, it needs movement and deep breathing to pump its fluid through the body and escort toxins out).

A special massage therapy known as lymph drainage, or lymphatic massage, is designed to help sluggish lymph fluid get moving. Trained therapists use hands-on techniques to detect the direction, strength, and quality of the lymph flow, then perform gentle massage movements to stimulate the pathways and improve the flow. To learn more about this therapy, check out www.vodderschool.com or www.upledger.com.

KICK ACID TIP #14

Massage Acids Out of Your Body

You can improve the flow of your lymphatic system through self-massage using any or all of the following pure essential oils: geranium, juniper, or black pepper. Simply add 3 drops of each to 3 tablespoons of a carrier oil (a gentle oil for "carrying" stronger medicinal essential oils) such as grapeseed, apricot kernel, almond, or olive oil. Mix in a small bowl, then rub on your arms and legs, using long upward strokes and moving toward your heart with each stroke. Geranium, juniper, and black pepper oils are particularly good at improving lymph flow. Can't find one of them? Simply use one or two of the others. To ensure that you aren't allergic or sensitive to these oils, be sure to do a patch test of the oil blend (not the straight essential oils) on your inner arm and wait 48 hours before rubbing the oil mixture over larger areas of your body.

Acupuncture and Acupressure

Acupuncture is one of the oldest and most widely used forms of medical treatment in the world. While most people recognize acupuncture's roots in traditional Chinese medicine, similar practices developed in India and among

Maori people in New Zealand. While its age is disputed, acupuncture has been practiced for at least 5,000 years and possibly up to 10,000 years.

The main focus of acupuncture is the life force or energy of the body, which acupuncturists call "chi," or "qi" (both are pronounced "chee"). Chi is also found in water, food, and air. Acupuncture is about balancing the body's chi for optimum health. The two main streams of this energy, called "yin" and "yang," become disrupted by toxins such as acidic foods and stress hormones. This disruption of energy flow results in what Western medicine defines as symptoms: pain, inflammation, and fatigue, to name a few.

According to a 2002 survey conducted by the National Institutes of Health, more than 8.2 million Americans have used acupuncture for the prevention of pain or other health problems.[7] It is effective at treating numerous ailments, from back pain and menstrual cramps to headaches and fibromyalgia. A study funded by the National Center for Complementary and Alternative Medicine demonstrated that acupuncture provides pain relief and improves function for people with osteoarthritis of the knee.[8] There are hundreds of scientific studies like this one outlining the incredible effectiveness of acupuncture.

Acupuncturists insert ultra-fine needles into specific points on the body, determined by the symptoms and the diagnosis. The points are found along energy channels within the body. (French researchers conducted an experiment to test the veracity of these energy pathways, and validated their existence.[9]) Most people barely feel the insertion. Those who simply cannot get past the idea of needles can opt for acupressure, a needle-less form of the same energy-balancing techniques.

While I have seen the benefits of acupuncture in many patients with many different health concerns, very little research has been conducted on its effectiveness at reducing acidity in the body. However, acupuncture's immune-boosting properties would certainly play a role in helping your body deal with the impact of a pH imbalance. Acupuncture also helps the body get rid of toxic buildup in the joints, organs, and tissues that may be disrupting the proper flow of energy. Equally important, acupuncture is an excellent stress-reduction tool. I anticipate that, over time, research will validate acupuncture's ability to help restore acid–alkaline balance.

While many different types of health practitioners perform acupuncture, if you're looking for hormone- and pH-balancing effects, you're better off choosing a practitioner who practices traditional Chinese acupuncture, not a Western version of it. These practitioners are skilled at finding and correcting imbalances.

Therapeutic Touch

The term "therapeutic touch" is used to mean a particular hands-on therapy, as well as the entire realm of hands-on techniques, such as Reiki, Touch for Health, Jin Shin Jyutsu, and some forms of Reconnective Healing. In addition to reducing stress and anxiety, therapeutic touch has been shown to have positive effects on many conditions linked to acidity in the body, including osteoarthritis, cancer, irritable bowel syndrome, and Alzheimer's-type dementia.[10] It can provide an increased sense of comfort and well-being, reduce pain, and in some cases improve symptoms and the condition itself. More study is required to validate the power of therapeutic touch as a treatment, either stand-alone or in combination with other healing therapies and medical treatments. But because therapeutic touch has no side effects and can help reduce stress, it is a welcome addition to the Kick Acid program, should you choose to incorporate it.

Biofeedback Therapy

The principles of biofeedback have been with us for many decades, but modern technology and increased understanding of energy and bioenergetic medicine have given particularly exciting new life to this healing technique. The latest form uses a device capable of sending millions of electrical signals into the body each second. These signals "read" the organs, tissues, and cells and send information back regarding "stresses" or anomalies. Because all living organisms are energy life forms, they give off energetic frequencies. Different organisms have different frequencies, so a liver cell will have a different signal than a brain cell. And a healthy liver cell will have a different frequency than an unhealthy, stressed, diseased liver cell. The biofeedback device receives this information as a measure of stress on our body. It can also determine the body's level of reactivity to possible stressors, such as allergens, pathogens, or nutritional deficiencies, as well as a host of other factors that can affect health. It can even help identify whether a pH imbalance is stressing your body.

Some forms of biofeedback can deliver therapies to help normalize stress responses, reintroducing your body to healthy tissue and organ signals and thereby pointing it in the right direction for optimum health.

A word of caution regarding biofeedback: beware the weekend workshop practitioner who has little or no training as a health practitioner outside of biofeedback therapy. While biofeedback is noninvasive and pain-free, it is analogous to surgery—the scalpel is only as good as the person using it. Years of health training are required to understand and interpret the information provided by the biofeedback machine. No one can obtain that level of understanding in a weekend course. However, in the hands of a qualified health professional, biofeedback can help pinpoint underlying stressors you may be overlooking, and the practitioner can target key therapies that will help restore health.

Sauna Therapy

From the Native civilizations across North America to the Scandinavian cultures of northern Europe, people worldwide recognize the health benefits of increasing body temperature. The First Peoples of North America are well known for their healing sweat lodges. You may not have access to a sweat lodge, but you can benefit from the modern technological version of it: the sauna. While there are benefits to steam saunas and other types of saunas, I recommend far infrared (FIR) saunas to my patients.

With a far infrared sauna, you won't be pouring water over hot rocks to create steam and moist heat. The high temperatures and humidity of steam saunas can put your cardiovascular system or lungs at risk. FIR saunas mimic nature by delivering radiant heat through ceramic infrared heaters. No hot stones, no water, no humidity, but plenty of sweat. The energy delivered by a FIR sauna creates a "sweat volume" that is two to three times greater than that generated by a conventional steam sauna. Because this is accomplished at a lower (and therefore less risky) temperature, heart rate and blood pressure concerns are greatly reduced. For comparison's sake, FIR saunas typically operate in the 110°F to 130°F range, while steam saunas can reach 180°F to 235°F. The result of sitting in a FIR sauna: more sweat, and more acidic toxins excreted through the skin, in less time.

The word "radiation" has negative connotations in our society, and we try to avoid all things radioactive (if we know what they are). Radiation certainly can be lethal (think of atomic radiation from a nuclear bomb blast) or damaging (think of ultraviolet radiation from the sun). But the sun also delivers healing, warm rays, or radiant heat. This is infrared radiation, a form of energy that heats objects directly (in other words, it does not heat the air in between). Infrared energy can penetrate up to 3 inches beneath the skin, promoting healing at a deep tissue level. Infrared radiation also appears to work energetically at the cellular level. It can improve metabolism and blood circulation in addition to raising our core body temperature. An increased body temperature can inhibit the growth of acid-creating pathogens.

Athletes use saunas to promote recovery from injuries or strenuous workouts. Saunas also increase heart rate without increasing blood pressure. But while FIR saunas can help your body burn additional calories at a rate consistent with fairly strenuous exercise, such as marathon running or squash, they are not an alternative to regular exercise.

Many firefighters have adopted FIR sauna sessions into their health regime. Firefighters are exposed to countless chemicals and toxins when battling blazes, and despite the best safety equipment, these substances enter their bodies. In the wake of the tragic events of 9/11, many firefighters who were at the World Trade Center collapse began intensive sauna programs to help them overcome the severe toxic effects. Reports showed that, following sauna treatments, white towels used to wipe away sweat were sometimes stained blue or other colors by the toxic compounds leaving the body through the skin.

Jumping into a sauna certainly won't make up for a highly acidic diet, but it can help get your body back on track when your diet has been less than perfect. It's also a great lifestyle addition for people suffering from chronic illness, because eliminating any toxins the body may be harboring improves body chemistry faster. Many people suffering from arthritis, fibromyalgia, headaches, and other health concerns have found pain relief or improvement in the healing rays of a FIR sauna.

I love my FIR sauna. I use it daily in the cold winter months, when I am less active, and two or three times a week in the summer. A 20- or 30-minute sauna can keep me warm for hours, even in the dead of winter. More importantly, it gets me sweating profusely, allowing toxins to be excreted through my skin. Because you can also lose minerals this way (just as when you exercise too long and too hard), it is critical to drink an extra 2 cups of alkaline water for each sauna session and include foods high in minerals and vitamins in your diet.

While a FIR sauna is not an essential part of the Ultimate pH Solution, I highly recommend trying one out if a health center or spa in your area offers it as a therapy. FIR sauna therapy generally runs between $20 and $50 per session, but many health centers offer package discounts for 10 or more sessions. If you can afford to purchase a FIR sauna (they run to $2,000 to $6,000, depending on the size and model you choose), it can be a great lifestyle addition. The units often look like small cabins constructed of cedar or oak. The dimensions vary, but FIR saunas typically accommodate one to six people. For more information, visit www.infraredsauna.net.

KICK ACID TIP #15

Bathe the Acid Away

Baking soda is both alkaline and alkaline-forming. It can help to quickly restore your body's natural balance when you've been exposed to excessive acid through stress or consumption of acid-forming foods. Note, however, that bathing in a baking soda bath increases your alkalinity only slightly and is not an antidote to a poor diet. Add 1 cup of baking soda to your bathwater and soak for 20 minutes. Add a few drops of pure eucalyptus essential oil to enhance your breathing and invigorate you, or a few drops of lavender essential oil to relax your body and improve your sleep. The baking soda will leave your skin feeling incredibly soft. Have an acid-balancing bath once a week.

THE ALKALIZING POWER OF AN ATTITUDE ADJUSTMENT

Having a positive attitude can profoundly change our life experiences. In addition to helping us cope more effectively with stress, finding the positive value in our experiences can help balance our body chemistry.

A Positive Outlook

No one has a positive attitude all the time, but the more you try to think positive, the more you'll be kicking acid and warding off disease. Stress hormones acidify our bodies, so lowering them improves body chemistry and overall health. Emotions such as happiness, optimism, and joy boost the immune system, according to research conducted at the Sackler School of Medicine at Tel Aviv University and published in the journal *Autoimmunity Reviews*.[11] In a long-term study of older men, scientists at Harvard's School of Public Health and the Department of Veterans Affairs found that older men who had high levels of optimism had a dramatically reduced risk of angina, non-fatal heart attack, and death from coronary heart disease compared to men who were more pessimistic.[12] Other research, conducted by the American Heart Association and published in the journal *Circulation*, showed that worry is associated with an increased risk of coronary heart disease.[13] So do your best to think of the glass as half full!

Gratitude

In our materialistic society, we are exposed to an average of between 285 and 305 ads per day (depending on whether you are male or female, respectively) trying to sell us the latest, greatest something-or-other. So we may be inclined to focus on things we want or need instead of what truly matters in our life. By shifting your focus to gratitude for the things you *have* and the people with whom you share life, you'll help reduce acidic stress hormones.

KICK ACID TIP #16

Keep a Gratitude Journal

A number of years ago, when I returned to school to study international trade, I met a lovely woman named Aurelia, an international lawyer. We immediately became friends, and one day after class we went to a local restaurant. She generously shared with me that she kept a gratitude journal. Every day, she wrote down 10 things she was grateful for, both little things and big things. After the last class, she told me she had included me in her journal because she was grateful we had met and become friends. I was so touched by her story and her willingness to share it that I still remember it a decade later.

As Aurelia did, each day (or as often as you can) write down 10 things you are grateful for. They might include friendships, kind words, a warm home, meeting a friendly person, and so much more. By focusing your attention on the positive aspects of your life, you'll be helping to restore hormonal balance to your body, which in turn helps restore alkaline balance.

PUTTING IT ALL TOGETHER

The Ultimate pH Solution diet and lifestyle is not a make-work project. It is a "make your body work better for you" project, to give you more energy and vitality and lessen your risk of developing the numerous health problems related to our modern way of living and eating. In the next chapter, you will find more than 50 recipes to get you started on delicious, nutritious alkaline or wise acid meals. You will probably save money on your grocery bill, because meat, processed foods, and treats are often the most expensive items at the supermarket. And you are paying for those items twice: with your money and your health.

I'm not a zealot with my diet, and I don't expect anyone else to be.

Perfection is not the goal here; consistency is a much better objective, and one that will lead to a strong foundation for your future diet and lifestyle.

The key to lasting change is to take it slow, gradually introducing new behaviors and building toward your new lifestyle. If you change one aspect of your diet or lifestyle every week, you will be amazed at how much better you feel in a year. You could try something like this:

- **Week 1:** Stop adding sugar to your food and beverages, and eliminate foods containing sugars. Use stevia as a sweetener.
- **Week 2:** Drink at least 12 glasses of water each day (preferably filtered and alkaline water; you can add alkalizing drops to filtered water). If you are suffering from health problems or are overweight, increase your alkaline water consumption to 20 cups a day.
- **Week 3:** Stop eating at fast-food restaurants.
- **Week 4:** Walk or meditate for 30 minutes a day.
- **Week 5:** Try a new vegetable.
- **Week 6:** Refrain from buying processed foods, soft drinks, or bottled juices when grocery shopping.
- **Week 7:** Try a new recipe from chapter 8 each day.
- **Week 8:** Eat a big salad with every dinner.
- **Week 9:** Eat meat only once a week, if at all.
- **Week 10:** Buy your personal hygiene products, laundry supplies, and household cleaning products at a reputable health food store.

You can follow this plan exactly as is, or you can adapt it to suit your personality, lifestyle, and health goals. Make simple changes such as these over the next 10 weeks, and you'll be well on your way to kicking acid for almost 20 percent of the year.

There are other lifestyle changes that are essential to the Ultimate pH Solution. If you smoke, it is imperative that you quit. There's no time like the present. If you drink—well, in the best-case scenario, you'd stop, but at least dramatically minimize your consumption. Some of the toughest acid habits to break are everyday addictions to sugar, breads, dairy products, and caffeine. As is the case with most addictions, going cold turkey can make you feel awful for a few days. That's because your body is detoxifying from the acidic poisons, and the pathogens that have been feeding on the acidic substances you've been consuming are now starving. Don't try to quit all your bad habits at once; the shock will be too much for your body. Instead, ease into the improvements gradually. As the poisons are expelled from your body and the pathogens die off, you will begin to feel better and better—probably better than you have felt in years.

For more advice on gentle, safe, and effective detoxification, read my book *The 4-Week Ultimate Body Detox Plan.*

WHAT TO DO WHEN YOU'VE FALLEN OFF THE WAGON

So you've slipped off the wagon. You're only human, and it can sometimes be difficult to adjust to a new way of living. As Ralph Waldo Emerson said, "Finish each day and be done with it. You have done what you could. Some blunders and absurdities no doubt crept in; forget them as soon as you can. Tomorrow is a new day; begin it well and serenely and with too high a spirit to be encumbered with your old nonsense."

A Day in the Life of an Acid-Kicker

Still think kicking acid is difficult? Let me show you how easy it can be, even on a workday:

- Wake up and have 2 cups of pure, alkaline water with the juice of a freshly squeezed lemon.
- Dry skin brush, shower, and get dressed.
- Prepare Blueberry Avocado Delight (page 139) and eat breakfast.
- Begin your workday (at the office or at home).
- Have a peppermint tea during your coffee break, and if you are hungry, eat some raw almonds (preferably organic and unsalted).
- Drink at least 3 cups of water before noon. (Avoid drinking more than ½ cup of any beverage with meals, as it will dilute your much-needed digestive enzymes. To ensure healthy digestion, stop drinking 20 minutes before a meal and begin again no sooner than an hour after a meal.)
- Have a large salad at lunch (add some avocado) and go for a walk. If you cannot get away, find a quiet space for some time alone.
- Drink another 3 cups of water and a large green drink in the afternoon (but not with lunch).
- Do some deep-breathing exercises at your desk or when you first arrive home. If you are driving home, take some deep breaths when you are stuck in traffic or at stoplights.

- Have another large salad and Vegetable Tagine (page 165) or Fajitas (page 162) for dinner. For a treat, try Chocolate Mousse (page 171). If possible, don't eat after seven or eight o'clock in the evening.
- Wait at least an hour for dinner to digest, then drink another cup or two of water.
- Consider a gentle yoga class or go for a walk with a friend or loved one. Talk about your day and your hopes and dreams.
- Write 10 things in your gratitude journal.

That doesn't sound too painful or difficult, does it? You'll be amazed at how quickly these simple changes become an essential part of your life. Instead of being addicted to sugar, stress, adrenaline rushes, conflict, or food additives, you will be addicted to feeling energetic, sleeping well at night, thinking clearly, and maintaining a balanced mood. Your body, your mind, and your spirit will feel strong in a way that can never be achieved with an acidic life-style. You'll understand on a personal level the value of kicking acid for life.

One Week's Kick Acid Meal Plan

Here is a sample eating plan that will help you kick acid out of your diet. Try it for a week and see how much better you feel. All of the recipes are included in chapter 8. And don't forget, there's no need to count calories when you're eating a variety of healthy foods such as vegetables and alkalizing fruit. Simply pay attention to your body's signals: when you feel full, stop eating; when you're hungry, eat! If it has been more than two to three hours since your last meal or snack, it's time to eat again. If you're hungry on this program, you're not doing it right! Also, don't forget to drink plenty of water and green drinks throughout each day.

Sunday
Breakfast: grapefruit and one slice of toasted *Amaranth Bread* (page 146) with *Michelle's Better Butter* (page 154)
Snack: *Blood-Alkalizing Juice* (page 141)
Lunch: greens with avocado slices, a handful of blueberries, and *Herb Dressing* (page 160)
Snack: a handful of raw unsalted almonds
Dinner: *Fajitas* (page 162) and greens

Monday

Breakfast: *Eggless Scramble* (page 140; make twice the recipe and save half for Wednesday)

Snack: one slice of *Amaranth Bread* (page 146) with *Herbed Soft Cheese* (page 153)

Lunch: one or two *Veggie Wraps* (page 166)

Snack: *Hummus* (page 152) and vegetable crudités

Dinner: *Carrot Apple Celery Juice* (page 142; juice the carrots first and place carrot pulp in an airtight container for tomorrow's *Tuna-less Salad Sandwiches*), *Vegetable Tagine* (page 165), and greens topped with bean sprouts and *Asian Vinaigrette* (page 159)

Tuesday

Breakfast: *Mango Pudding* (page 139) and *Curt's Carrot Apple Whole Juice* (page 144)

Snack: grapefruit

Lunch: *Tuna-less Salad Sandwiches* (page 165)

Snack: *Hummus* (page 152) and vegetable crudités

Dinner: *Bobbi's Caesar Salad* (page 158), and a slice or two of *Herb Spelt Bread* (page 147)

Wednesday

Breakfast: *Kick Acid Citrus Cleanser* (page 144) and *Eggless Scramble* (page 140)

Snack: a handful of raw unsalted almonds

Lunch: greens with *Sesame Sensation Dressing* (page 161), *Salsa Fresca* (page 151), and homemade *Tortilla Chips* (page 150)

Snack: slice of *Herb Spelt Bread* (page 147) with *Michelle's Better Butter* (page 154)

Dinner: *Red Pepper–Butternut Squash Quesadillas* (page 163) served with *Herbed Soft Cheese* (page 153) for dipping

Thursday

Breakfast: grapefruit and one slice of toasted *Amaranth Bread* (page 146) with *Michelle's Better Butter* (page 154)

Snack: *Hummus* (page 152) and vegetable crudités

Lunch: *Winter Vegetable Soup* (page 156) and homemade *Tortilla Chips* (page 150)

Snack: celery sticks filled with *Mom's Omega-3 Almond Butter* (page 154)

Dinner: Mexican salad made of greens topped with *Salsa Fresca* (page 151) and *Guacamole* (page 152), served with *Tortilla Chips* (page 150)

Friday

Breakfast: *Blueberry Avocado Delight* (page 139), and one slice of toasted *Amaranth Bread* (page 146) served with *Mom's Omega-3 Almond Butter* (page 154)

Snack: grapefruit

Lunch: greens with bean sprouts, rice noodles, and *Asian Vinaigrette* (page 159), topped with chopped fresh cilantro and coarsely chopped raw almonds

Snack: an apple

Dinner: *Bobbi's Green Grasshopper* (page 142), green salad with *Sesame Sensation Dressing* (page 161), and *Vegetable Tagine* (page 165)

Dessert: *Chocolate Mousse* (page 171)

Saturday

Breakfast: *Sweet Potato Hash Browns* (page 140), one slice of toasted *Amaranth Bread* (page 146) served with *Michelle's Better Butter* (page 154), and *Kick Acid Citrus Cleanser* (page 144)

Snack: grapefruit

Lunch: *Roasted Carrot Soup* (page 155) and *Tabbouleh Salad* (page 159)

Snack: a handful of raw unsalted almonds

Dinner: *Slow Cooker Black Bean Chili* (page 164) with a dollop of *Guacamole* (page 152) and *Southwestern Bruschetta* (page 150)

pH SOLUTION

Kirk Turns Off His Flu Magnet

Kirk, a gentle and kind man in his early 30s, told me he was "tired of getting every cold and flu that's going around." Because he was surrounded by many co-workers at his government job, he was exposed to every germ that arrived at work along with his colleagues. For him, there was no "season" for flu: germs were present at his office year-round. Kirk had six or seven viral infections every year, and his medical doctor simply told him that was "normal." But Kirk didn't agree. He said, "If six or seven infections per year is normal, I don't want to be normal any more." He asked if it was possible for him to build up his immune system so he wouldn't constantly fall prey to germs and bacteria.

"It's more than possible—it's a sure thing," I told him. I explained that viruses can survive only in an acidic environment. When your blood becomes too acidic, viruses thrive. Conversely, if your blood is alkalized, viruses die. Acid to a virus is like oxygen to a human being. Remove acidity from your body and viruses will die or find someone else's body to inhabit.

We reviewed his diet. Though Kirk considered himself a healthy eater, his diet was quite acidic, leaving him vulnerable to viruses and bacteria. He drank at least 3 cups of milk a day "to get enough calcium," drank sugary fruit punch instead of water, ate some form of animal protein at almost every meal, and ate dessert after most meals. He did eat a decent amount of vegetables at lunch and dinner.

Kirk decided to give a more alkaline diet a try and was astonished by the results. He has stayed on it for five years, and during that time, the one brief flu he had came during his Christmas holidays, when he "ate too much junk." Happily, this one departure from full-time health only served to strengthen his intent to return to alkalinity and stay there. Since resuming his alkaline-boosting program, he has remained healthy and flu- and virus-free.

CHAPTER 8

Kick Acid Recipes to Delight the Palate

"If more of us valued food and cheer and song above hoarded gold, it would be a merrier world."

—J.R.R. TOLKIEN

This chapter is packed with delicious, nutritious, alkalizing recipes to help you stay healthy for life. Eating a more alkaline diet to maximize healing, disease prevention, and balanced weight is easier than you might think. A predominantly alkaline diet includes lots of vegetables and smaller amounts of certain grains, nuts, legumes, and fruit, prepared in dishes that help your body restore balance without sacrificing taste. Some of these recipes are among my favorites—and trust me, I love great-tasting gourmet foods. Do not let their healthy nature put you off. Keep an open mind as you learn about new preparation techniques and foods you might not have given a second thought to. You will discover real treasures among them, and I am sure some of these recipes will become your favorites too.

You'll find recipes that are terrific substitutes for common items in your diet. Recipes such as Michelle's Better Butter (page 154), Almond Milk (page 145), and Yam Fries (page 167) have all the taste of your favorite foods, without the acidity!

Not all of these recipes are alkalizing to the body. For example, I've included a few desserts, but they are healthier options than the extremely acid-forming desserts most people eat. Remember that we're not trying to eat a completely alkaline diet; rather, we're aiming to stay within the 70:30 ratio of alkaline to acidic foods.

...es a great substitute for acid-forming eggs and is loaded with ...d fiber from the vegetables, as well as lean protein and calcium from ...alizing tofu. It's perfect for breakfast or as a quick dinner. Turmeric, a spice ...mmonly used in Indian cooking, is a natural anti-inflammatory.

> 8 oz firm tofu, crumbled
> 1 tsp ground turmeric
> 1 tsp Celtic sea salt
> ½ tsp ground cumin (optional)
> 4 tomatoes, quartered
> 2 tbsp extra-virgin olive oil
> 1 large onion, chopped
> 1 small sweet potato, chopped (optional)
> 2 stalks celery, chopped
> 1 red bell pepper, chopped

1. In a bowl, combine tofu, turmeric, salt, and cumin; set aside.
2. In a blender or food processor, purée tomatoes; set aside.
3. In a large skillet, heat oil over medium-low heat, making sure it never smokes. Sauté onion until softened. Add sweet potato (if using) and sauté until tender. Add celery and red pepper; sauté until tender. Add seasoned tofu and sauté until heated through. Stir in tomato purée, cover, and cook for 5 to 10 minutes, or until tomato purée is heated through and flavors have blended.

SWEET POTATO HASH BROWNS

A terrific breakfast option, these hash browns also make a satisfying snack or side dish when you have a craving for something salty.

> 3 tbsp extra-virgin olive oil
> 1 large onion, chopped
> 3 sweet potatoes or yams, cubed
> Celtic sea salt or Himalayan salt

1. In a large skillet, heat oil over medium-low heat, making sure it never smokes. Sauté onion and sweet potatoes for 20 to 30 minutes, or until onions are golden-brown and sweet potato is soft. Season with salt to taste.

BREAKFAST

While I've listed these recipes as break[...] any time of day. Some of them make [...] make nutritious desserts.

BLUEBERRY AVOCADO DELIGHT

This recipe is quick and easy to prepare and can b[...] [...]reakfast or a delectable dessert.

> 1 avocado, peeled and pitted
> Juice of ½ lemon
> 1 cup frozen blueberries

1. In a food processor, purée avocado, lemon juice, and ½ cup of the blueberries until smooth (or use a hand blender). Top with the remaining blueberries and serve immediately.

Variation

Add ¼ cup coarsely chopped nuts (such as unsalted raw almonds) for a yummy fruit and nut treat.

MANGO PUDDING   SERVES 2 TO 4

Mango pudding makes a fantastic breakfast or dessert. While the mango is acid-forming, the avocado is alkaline-forming. The recipe as a whole is neutral to slightly acidic, and is loaded with healthy nutrients and essential fatty acids.

> 1 to 2 mangos, peeled, pitted, and chopped
> 1 avocado, peeled and pitted

1. In a food processor, purée mangos and avocado until smooth (or use a hand blender). Serve immediately.

Tip: Mangos turn yellowish when they are ripe. When avocados are ripe, their skin turns blackish and yields slightly when pressed with a fingertip.

The Ultimate pH Solution

EGGLESS SCRAMB[...]

This dish mak[...]
nutrients a[...]
the al[...]
c[...]

140

BEVERAGES

There are two main types of juice you can make: extracts and total juices. Extracts are made in a traditional juicer, which extracts the juice from the fibrous part of fruits and vegetables. Total juices are made in a high-power blender, and the whole fruit or vegetable is liquefied with some added water, giving you both the juice and the fiber from the foods. (For more information on juicers and high-power blenders, see Resources, page 182.)

There are nutritional benefits to both types. The nutrients from extracts are quickly absorbed into your bloodstream, giving you a boost of energy and lots of vitamins and minerals. Total juices are absorbed more slowly, thanks to the fiber, which helps to keep your blood sugar levels stable while the vitamins and minerals are absorbed into your blood. As a bonus, total juices increase your fiber intake, keeping your intestinal tract cleansed from acidic toxins.

In this section, I've included recipes for seven extracts and one total juice, as well as a spritzer and a milk substitute. Enjoy!

BLOOD-ALKALIZING JUICE   SERVES 1

Not just a garden pest, dandelion is loaded with alkaline minerals that remove acidic toxins from the blood, tissues, joints, and kidneys. Be aware that if you drink a fair amount of this juice over a short period of time, it can speed up a cleansing reaction, which might initially produce symptoms such as fatigue or headaches. These will pass as your body becomes "cleaner."

> 2 apples, cored
> 1 cucumber
> Large handful fresh dandelion greens

1. In a juicer, juice apples, cucumber, and dandelion greens. Pour over ice and drink immediately.

Tip: If you dig the dandelion greens yourself, be sure to find organic dandelion from an area where the land hasn't been sprayed with pesticides for several years and that is far removed from traffic. Dandelion greens are also available in many grocery stores and markets, particularly fruit and vegetable markets.

BOBBI'S GREEN GRASSHOPPER   SERVES 1 TO 2

Don't be put off by the wheatgrass in this recipe: it is full of minerals and is extremely alkalizing. The carrots and apples transform it into a delicious juice.

   8 carrots, tops removed
   2 apples, cored
   1 cup wheatgrass

1. In a juicer, juice carrots, apples, and wheatgrass. Pour over ice and drink immediately.

Tip: Wheatgrass is available at many health food stores.

CARROT APPLE CELERY JUICE   SERVES 1

This tasty juice is also powerful medicine—it's packed with beta carotene from the carrots, and the celery contributes over 20 anti-pain and anti-inflammatory compounds.

   4 carrots, tops removed
   2 stalks celery
   1 apple, cored

1. In a juicer, juice carrots, celery, and apple. Pour over ice and drink immediately.

CARROT APPLE GINGER JUICE   SERVES 1

This sounds like an odd combination of ingredients, but is absolutely fantastic. It's my favorite juice. It is high in natural sugar from the carrots and apple, so is best diluted 1:1 with pure water. If you're suffering from pain of any kind, ginger is a marvelous natural pain remedy.

   6 large carrots, tops removed
   1 apple, cored
   1-inch piece gingerroot

1. In a juicer, juice carrots, apple, and ginger. Pour over ice and drink immediately.

SUE'S VEGGIE JUICE   SERVES 4

When my copyeditor, Sue Sumeraj, is not busy working her magic on books, she can often be found making this fantastic and highly nutritious juice, which she agreed to share. Don't be put off by its swamp-water-like appearance—it tastes far better than it looks. And what a powerhouse of nutrients!

> 1 green apple, cored
> 4 carrots, tops removed
> 3 stalks celery
> 1 red bell pepper
> ½ cucumber
> Large handful spinach
> 1-inch piece gingerroot

1. In a juicer, juice apple, carrots, celery, red pepper, cucumber, spinach, and ginger. Pour over ice and drink immediately.

ANTI-PAIN, ANTI-INFLAMMATORY JUICE   SERVES 1

Celery is full of alkalizing minerals, as well as more than 20 compounds that reduce pain and inflammation.

> 4 stalks celery
> 1 cucumber
> 1 apple, cored

1. In a juicer, juice celery, cucumber, and apple. Pour over ice and drink immediately.

INSTANT ALKALIZER JUICE   SERVES 1

The cucumber in this juice is loaded with alkaline minerals that help restore your body's biochemistry quickly. The beets, greens, and carrots make it a nutritional powerhouse.

> 3 carrots, tops removed
> 1 cucumber
> ½ beet, with greens

1. In a juicer, juice carrots, cucumber, and beet. Pour over ice and drink immediately.

KICK ACID CITRUS CLEANSER   SERVES 1

This juice can be made with a fruit and vegetable juicer, a citrus juicer, or a high-power blender, whichever you prefer.

    1 grapefruit
    ½ lemon
    1 cup purified alkaline water
    Powdered stevia (optional)

1. In a juicer or high-power blender, juice grapefruit, lemon, and water. Sweeten with stevia to taste, if desired. Pour over ice and drink immediately.

CURT'S CARROT APPLE WHOLE JUICE   SERVES 2

Need a blast of fiber to get things moving, while satisfying a sweet craving? Try my husband's quick and simple total juice. Unlike extracts, it provides all the fiber—and it tastes great too!

    2 carrots, cut into 1-inch chunks
    1 apple, cored and quartered
    2 cups purified alkaline water (or more if you prefer a thinner juice)
    1 tsp cherry powder (optional)
    1 tsp blueberry powder (optional)

1. In a high-power blender, blend carrots, apple, water, and cherry and blueberry powders (if using) until smooth. Drink immediately, before juice starts to thicken.

Tip: Cherry and blueberry powder are available at many health food stores. Be sure they have no sweeteners or artificial ingredients.

APPLE-BERRY SPRITZER   SERVES 2 TO 4

A much healthier option than soda pop, this spritzer contains fruit juice, which is acidic, as well as alkalizing baking soda to add fizz. Drink only in moderation.

    1 cup pure, unsweetened, preservative-free fruit juice
    1 cup purified water
    1 tsp baking soda

1. In a pitcher, combine fruit juice, water, and baking soda, stirring to dissolve the baking soda.

Tip: I use Ceres apple berry juice, found in small cartons in most grocery stores.

ALMOND MILK   SERVES 2 TO 4

Drink almond milk on its own, or use it as a base for fruit smoothies or in baking recipes.

    2 cups purified alkaline water
    ½ cup unsalted raw almonds
    8 drops liquid stevia (add more drops for a sweeter almond milk)

1. In a blender, blend water, almonds, and stevia until smooth. Strain, if desired.

Tip: Liquid stevia can be found in most health food stores.

BREAD AND BUNS

My husband loves bread so much that I call him a "bread head." Bread was the one food he didn't want to give up when he changed his eating habits. But the main ingredients in most breads are acidic, from the white or whole wheat flour to the sugar, shortening, and yeast. So I spent hours in the kitchen developing some delicious bread recipes that are free of unhealthy ingredients and are slightly alkalizing to neutral. All of these breads have spelt flour as their primary ingredient. Spelt is an ancient grain in the same family as wheat, but, unlike wheat, it hasn't been hybridized to become severely acid-forming. It is one of the few alkaline-forming grains. The psyllium in these recipes is an excellent high-fiber stand-in for acid-forming eggs.

With these amazing recipes, you can have your bread and eat it too—and still be kicking acid. Serve thick slices with Michelle's Better Butter (page 154) for a tasty and nutritious snack, appetizer, or addition to any meal.

AMARANTH BREAD   SERVES 8 TO 10

Amaranth Bread is an all-purpose bread that works well for sandwiches and toast. Serve it topped with Michelle's Better Butter or Mom's Omega-3 Almond Butter (page 154).

> 3 cups spelt flour
> ½ cup amaranth flour
> 2 tsp ground psyllium hulls
> 1½ tsp baking soda
> 1 tsp Celtic sea salt
> ¼ tsp powdered stevia
> 3 cups Almond Milk (see recipe, page 145)
> ½ cup organic extra-virgin coconut oil

1. Preheat oven to 350ºF and grease an 8- by 4-inch loaf pan with extra-virgin coconut oil or olive oil.

2. In a food processor or mixer, combine spelt flour, amaranth flour, psyllium, baking soda, salt, and stevia. Add Almond Milk and coconut oil; process until smooth.

3. Pour into prepared pan and bake for 75 minutes, or until a toothpick inserted in the center of the loaf comes out clean. Let cool in pan on a wire rack for 5 to 10 minutes before slicing.

Tip: Ground psyllium hulls (or husks, as they are sometimes called) are available at most health food stores, as are the other less common ingredients in this recipe.

HERB SPELT BREAD   SERVES 8 TO 10

This is my husband's favorite bread, and that's saying a lot.

    3½ cups spelt flour
    2 tsp ground psyllium hulls (see tip, above)
    1½ tsp baking soda
    1 tsp Celtic sea salt
    3 cups Almond Milk (see recipe, page 145)
    ½ cup organic extra-virgin coconut oil
    ½ cup finely chopped fresh herbs (such as basil, thyme, oregano,
        rosemary, chives) and/or green onions

1. Preheat oven to 350ºF and grease an 8- by 4-inch loaf pan with extra-virgin coconut oil or olive oil.

2. In a food processor or mixer, combine spelt flour, psyllium, baking soda, and salt. Add Almond Milk and coconut oil; process until smooth. Add herbs and process briefly until evenly dispersed.

3. Pour into prepared pan and bake for 75 minutes, or until a toothpick inserted in the center of the loaf comes out clean. Let cool in pan on a wire rack for 5 to 10 minutes before slicing.

Tip: When you're preparing a baked goods recipe that calls for eggs, replace each egg with 1 tsp ground psyllium hulls and 2 tbsp water. Or use 1 tsp ground flaxseeds and 2 tbsp water.

ZUCCHINI BREAD   SERVES 8 TO 10

This sweet bread makes a scrumptious dessert loaf or pairs well with an afternoon herbal tea. It's one of my favorites.

    3½ cups spelt flour
    2 tsp ground psyllium hulls (see tip, page 147)
    1½ tsp baking soda
    1 tsp Celtic sea salt
    ½ tsp powdered stevia
    ½ tsp ground cinnamon
    ¼ tsp ground cloves
    ¼ tsp ground ginger
    Pinch ground nutmeg
    2 cups Almond Milk (see recipe, page 145)
    ½ cup organic extra-virgin coconut oil
    1 cup grated zucchini

1. Preheat oven to 350ºF and grease an 8- by 4-inch loaf pan with extra-virgin coconut oil or olive oil.

2. In a food processor or mixer, combine spelt flour, psyllium, baking soda, salt, stevia, cinnamon, cloves, ginger, and nutmeg. Add Almond Milk and coconut oil; process until smooth. Add zucchini and process briefly until evenly dispersed.

3. Pour into prepared pan and bake for 75 minutes, or until a toothpick inserted in the center of the loaf comes out clean. Let cool in pan on a wire rack for 5 to 10 minutes before slicing.

Tip: When you're preparing a baked goods recipe that calls for baking powder, replace each 1 tsp baking powder with ½ tsp baking soda.

ZUCCHINI THYME DINNER BUNS   MAKES 12 BUNS

These savory buns are the perfect accompaniment to salads, soups, stews, or chili.

3½ cups spelt flour
1½ tsp baking soda
1 tsp Celtic sea salt
2 cups Almond Milk (see recipe, page 145)
½ cup extra-virgin olive oil
1 cup grated zucchini
1 green onion, finely chopped
Handful fresh basil leaves, finely chopped
1 tbsp finely chopped fresh thyme (leaves only)
Additional Celtic sea salt

1. Preheat oven to 350ºF and grease a 12-cup muffin tin with extra-virgin olive oil (or line with unbleached paper liners).

2. In a food processor or mixer, combine spelt flour, baking soda, and salt. Add Almond Milk and olive oil; process until smooth. Add zucchini, green onion, basil, and thyme; process briefly until evenly dispersed.

3. Spoon evenly into prepared muffin cups and sprinkle tops with a small amount of salt. Bake for 25 minutes, or until a toothpick inserted in the center of a bun comes out clean. Let cool in pan on a wire rack for 5 to 10 minutes.

APPETIZERS, DIPS, AND SPREADS

You can still enjoy great-tasting snacks and appetizers while you're kicking acid out of your body. Here are some fabulous recipes for bruschetta, salsa, guacamole, tortilla chips, and more.

SOUTHWESTERN BRUSCHETTA   SERVES 2 TO 4

Here's a Mexican twist on an Italian favorite. I could eat this almost daily—it's that good. And it's easy to prepare for a snack, appetizer, or quick lunch.

    4 to 6 slices sprouted-grain bread or yeast-free spelt or brown rice bread
    1 clove garlic
    Avocado Salsa (see recipe, page 151)

1. Toast bread until fairly crisp. Rub each slice with garlic. Place on serving dishes and top with Avocado Salsa. Serve immediately.

TORTILLA CHIPS   SERVES 4 TO 6

Healthier and more alkalizing than store-bought tortilla chips, this tasty alternative can be eaten on its own as a snack or as an accompaniment to soup, salad, or chili. Serve with Salsa Fresca (page 151), Avocado Salsa (page 151), Guacamole (page 152), or Hummus (page 152).

    1 package sprouted-grain or brown rice tortillas
    Extra-virgin olive oil
    Celtic sea salt or Himalayan salt

1. Preheat oven to 350°F. Place tortillas in a single layer on baking sheets, brush with a small amount of olive oil, and sprinkle with salt. Bake for 5 to 10 minutes, or until lightly browned. Break into chips and serve.

SALSA FRESCA   SERVES 2 TO 4

Think you don't have time to make fresh salsa? Think again. This nutritious recipe can be whipped up in minutes. Serve with Tortilla Chips (page 150).

> 1 clove garlic
> 2 green onions, cut into 2-inch pieces
> Large handful fresh cilantro
> 5 plum (Roma) tomatoes, halved
> Juice of 1 lime
> 1 tsp ground psyllium hulls (optional)
> ½ tsp Celtic sea salt or Himalayan salt
> Pinch cayenne pepper

1. In a food processor, process garlic until finely minced. Add green onions and cilantro; process until coarsely chopped. Add tomatoes, lime juice, psyllium (if using), salt, and cayenne; pulse until coarsely chopped.

Tip: The optional psyllium will help thicken the salsa.

Make ahead: Store in an airtight container in the refrigerator for up to 3 days.

AVOCADO SALSA   SERVES 2 TO 4

Serve with Tortilla Chips (page 150) or on toasted sprouted-grain bread or yeast-free spelt bread.

> 1 clove garlic
> Large handful fresh cilantro
> 2 large tomatoes, quartered
> Juice of 1 lime or lemon
> Pinch Celtic sea salt or Himalayan salt
> Pinch cayenne pepper
> 1 avocado, peeled, pitted, and cubed

1. In a food processor, process garlic until finely minced. Add cilantro and process until coarsely chopped. Add tomatoes, lime juice, salt, and cayenne; pulse until coarsely chopped.
2. Transfer to a serving bowl, add avocado, and toss gently to combine.

GUACAMOLE   SERVES 2 TO 4

Serve as a dip with Tortilla Chips (page 150) or carrot sticks, celery sticks, sliced red or green pepper, and broccoli or cauliflower florets. Or use as a spread on wraps and sandwiches. Use soon after making, or the guacamole will discolor.

    1 avocado, peeled and pitted
    Juice of ½ lime
    1 tbsp organic cold-pressed flaxseed oil
    Pinch Celtic sea salt

1. In a food processor, purée avocado, lime juice, flaxseed oil, and salt until smooth (or use a hand blender).

Variation
Garlic Guacamole: Add 1 clove of garlic with the avocado.

HUMMUS   SERVES 4 TO 6

Serve as a dip with Tortilla Chips (page 150) or crudités. Or use as a spread on wraps and sandwiches.

    2 cups cooked chickpeas (see page 171 for cooking instructions)
    ¼ cup chopped fresh parsley
    Juice of 1 lemon
    1 large clove garlic (or 2 small)
    ¼ tsp ground cumin

1. In a food processor, purée chickpeas, parsley, lemon juice, garlic, and cumin until smooth.

Make ahead: Store in an airtight container in the refrigerator for up to 1 week.

Variation
For a creamier hummus, add 1 to 2 tbsp of extra-virgin olive oil. Add gradually through the feed tube with the motor running, after the other ingredients are puréed.

ROASTED GARLIC SPREAD   MAKES ABOUT ½ CUP

Use as a spread on wraps and sandwiches, serve as a dip with Tortilla Chips (page 150) or crudités, or add to dressings, soups, and sauces.

> 1 large head garlic
> Extra-virgin olive oil

1. Preheat oven to 350ºF.
2. Slice the top off the garlic head, exposing the top of each clove. Place in a small baking dish (or on a sheet of foil). Drizzle with a small amount of olive oil and cover (or wrap). Bake for 45 to 60 minutes, or until garlic is tender. Let cool, then scoop cloves into a small bowl and mash.

Make ahead: Store in an airtight container in the refrigerator for up to 1 week.

HERBED SOFT CHEESE   MAKES ABOUT 2 CUPS

Similar to ricotta, savory cream cheese, or soft goat's cheese, this cheese has all the taste but none of the acidity of dairy cheeses. Also, it's high in usable calcium. It can be used to make vegetarian lasagna and other recipes that call for a soft cheese. It also makes a great dip for vegetables or Tortilla Chips (page 150), and a terrific sandwich spread.

> 3 tbsp extra-virgin olive oil
> 1 large onion, chopped
> 1 lb firm tofu
> Juice of 1 lemon
> 1 tsp Celtic sea salt or Himalayan salt
> 1 tsp unpasteurized honey
> 2 tbsp chopped fresh herbs (such as basil, oregano, thyme, rosemary)
>   and/or roasted garlic

1. In a skillet, heat 1 tbsp of the oil over medium-low heat, making sure it never smokes. Sauté onion for 10 to 15 minutes, or until lightly browned.
2. In a food processor, purée tofu, lemon juice, salt, honey, and the remaining oil until smooth. Add onion and process until combined.
3. Transfer to a serving bowl and stir in herbs.

Make ahead: Prepare through Step 2 and store in an airtight container for up to 4 days. Add herbs just before serving.

MICHELLE'S BETTER BUTTER
MAKES ABOUT 1 CUP

Serve this soft, healthier butter substitute on warm Herb Spelt Bread (page 147) or any other bread recipe.

½ cup organic extra-virgin coconut oil
½ cup organic cold-pressed flaxseed oil

1. In a small saucepan, over low heat, liquefy coconut oil. Immediately remove from heat and add flaxseed oil, stirring until well mixed. Pour into a serving container and refrigerate until firm.

Make ahead: Store in an airtight container in the refrigerator for up to 6 months.

Variation
Michelle's Better Basil Butter: Immediately after adding the flaxseed oil, stir in a handful of chopped fresh basil.

MOM'S OMEGA-3 ALMOND BUTTER
MAKES ABOUT 2½ CUPS

My mom created this fantastic alkalizing recipe to get more omega-3 fatty acids in her diet. It can be spread on sprouted-grain or spelt bread for breakfast or lunch, or spread on celery sticks for a snack.

3 cups unsalted raw almonds
½ cup organic cold-pressed flaxseed oil

1. In a food processor, coarsely chop almonds. With the motor running, through the feed tube, slowly add flaxseed oil; process until smooth.

Make ahead: Store in an airtight container in the refrigerator for up to 6 months.

SOUPS

Meals don't have to be complex. Sometimes, a quick and easy soup makes the perfect meal.

GAZPACHO	SERVES 2 TO 4

No cooking and lots of nutrients—what could be better? This fabulous soup can be whipped up in minutes, and you'll benefit from plentiful amounts of enzymes that would be destroyed by cooking.

> 5 tomatoes, quartered
> 1-inch slice cucumber, peeled
> ½ tsp Celtic sea salt or Himalayan salt
> Pinch cayenne pepper
> Small handful fresh cilantro, finely chopped
> 2 green onions, finely chopped

1. In a blender or food processor, purée tomatoes, cucumber, salt, and cayenne until smooth. Pour into serving bowls and sprinkle with cilantro and green onions.

ROASTED CARROT SOUP	SERVES 2 TO 4

This tasty soup is fast and easy to prepare, and it's alkalizing too.

> 2 tbsp extra-virgin olive oil
> 1½ onions, chopped
> 6 to 8 carrots, chopped
> 2½ cups purified alkaline water
> 1½ tsp ground cumin
> 1 tsp vegetable salt or Celtic sea salt
> Pinch cayenne pepper

1. In a large skillet, heat oil over medium-low heat, making sure it never smokes. Sauté onions and carrots for 10 to 15 minutes, or until golden brown.

2. Transfer to a blender or food processor and add water, cum enne; purée until smooth. Serve immediately.

Variation
If you prefer a thinner soup, add more water. You may wish to ings accordingly.

WINTER VEGETABLE SOUP   SERVES 2 TO 4

This easy, creamy soup is perfect when you want something warm and soothing on a cold winter night but don't have a lot of energy or desire to cook. It takes about an hour or so for the vegetables to roast, but the preparation time is only about 5 minutes.

3 carrots, cut into ¼-inch-thick slices
2 sweet potatoes, cut into ½-inch-thick slices
2 cloves garlic
1 small rutabaga (or ½ large), cut into ½-inch-thick slices
1 large onion, cut into large chunks
3 tbsp extra-virgin olive oil
1 tbsp dried basil
1 tsp ground cumin
½ tsp vegetable salt
¼ tsp cayenne pepper (or to taste)
Pinch ground nutmeg
2 cups purified alkaline water

1. Preheat oven to 350°F.

2. In a large bowl, combine carrots, sweet potatoes, garlic, rutabaga, and onion. Drizzle with olive oil and sprinkle with basil, cumin, salt, cayenne, and nutmeg. Toss to coat vegetables evenly.

3. Spread vegetables in a thin layer on a baking sheet (or 2 baking sheets, if necessary). Roast for 50 to 60 minutes, or until tender and lightly browned.

4. Transfer to a blender or food processor and add water; purée until smooth.

Tip: Rutabagas are roundish root vegetables. The skin is mostly white or cream-colored, with a hint of purple. Cut the outer skin off to reveal a firm, golden vegetable inside.

Variation
If you prefer a thinner soup, add more water. You may wish to adjust the seasonings accordingly.

SALADS AND SALAD DRESSINGS

Try to eat a large raw salad daily. Eat cooked food, such as baked sweet potatoes, cooked millet, or steamed or sautéed salmon, as an accompaniment. Once you make this eating pattern habitual, it is actually quite simple. Alternatively, place salad ingredients on a sprouted-grain or brown rice tortilla to turn it into a delicious wrap.

Salads don't have to be the boring things most people make them out to be. There are a tremendous number of delectable salads you can make if you vary the ingredients. Below is a list of possible ingredients to help you get started. While some of the options are slightly acid-forming, used in moderation their effects will be tempered if you use greens and/or sprouts as the primary ingredient. Be creative!

- mixed greens (mesclun), Boston lettuce, leaf lettuce, romaine lettuce, radicchio
- pea shoots, alfalfa sprouts, broccoli sprouts, clover sprouts, mung bean sprouts, onion sprouts
- chickpeas (garbanzo beans), Great Northern beans, kidney beans, lima beans, pinto beans, other legumes
- apples, avocados, blueberries, grapefruit, olives, oranges, raspberries, strawberries
- bell peppers, broccoli, cabbage, carrots, celery, cucumbers, mushrooms (raw or cooked), peas, green onions
- edible flowers
- cilantro, parsley, basil

BOBBI'S CAESAR SALAD   SERVES 4

My sister shared one of her favorite recipes for Caesar salad. This version is alkalizing and is made with beneficial fats that support healthy immune system and brain functions.

> 1 head romaine lettuce, torn into bite-sized pieces

Croutons

> 4 slices sprouted-grain bread, broken into bite-sized pieces
> 2 cloves garlic, finely chopped
> 2 tbsp extra-virgin olive oil
> 1 tsp dried basil
> 1 tsp dried thyme
> 1 tsp dried oregano

Dressing

> 2 to 3 cloves garlic
> 2 stalks celery, cut into 2-inch pieces
> Juice of 2 lemons
> 2 tbsp miso
> 1 cup organic cold-pressed flaxseed oil
> 1 cup extra-virgin olive oil

1. Preheat oven to 300°F.

2. Prepare the croutons: Spread bread in a single layer on a baking sheet and bake until crisp, about 10 to 20 minutes depending on the size of the croutons.

3. Meanwhile, in a large bowl, combine garlic, oil, basil, thyme, and oregano. Add baked bread pieces and toss to coat.

4. Prepare the dressing: In a food processor, process garlic, celery, lemon juice, and miso until celery is finely chopped. With the motor running, through the feed tube, gradually add flaxseed oil and olive oil; process until smooth.

5. Place romaine in a large serving bowl. Pour in dressing to taste and toss to coat. (Refrigerate remaining dressing for up to one week.) Top with croutons.

Variations

For a delicate alternative, use red leaf lettuce instead of romaine.
If you want to increase the tart taste of the dressing, use 3 lemons.

TABBOULEH SALAD

SERVES 2 AS AN ENTRÉE

Popular in Middle Eastern and Mediterranean countries, tabb made with acidic wheat couscous. This version is very alka quinoa, lemon juice, and parsley. The recipe is quick and easy to prepare, but the flavors deepen after it sits in the fridge for an hour or two.

2 tomatoes, chopped
1 large bunch fresh parsley (or 2 small bunches), finely chopped
1 clove garlic, finely chopped
1 green onion, chopped
2 cups cooked quinoa (see page 172 for cooking instructions)
Juice of 3 lemons
2 tbsp extra-virgin olive oil
½ tsp Celtic sea salt or Himalayan salt
Pinch cayenne pepper

1. In a large bowl, combine tomatoes, parsley, garlic, green onion, and quinoa.
2. In a separate bowl, whisk together lemon juice, olive oil, salt, and cayenne. Pour over salad and toss to coat.

Make ahead: Store in an airtight container in the refrigerator for up to 4 days. The flavors will mingle, making the salad taste even better.

ASIAN VINAIGRETTE

MAKES ABOUT 1½ CUPS

The rice vinegar and honey make this dressing acidic, but a large plate of greens balances the effects if you are moderate in your use of the dressing.

1 cup extra-virgin olive oil
½ cup rice vinegar
2 heaping tsp red miso
1 tsp unpasteurized honey

1. Place oil, vinegar, miso, and honey in a jar. Cover jar tightly and shake to blend (or use a hand blender).

Tip: Look for rice vinegar without preservatives, available at most health food stores.

Make ahead: Store in an airtight container in the refrigerator for up to 1 week.

UEBERRY DRESSING

While this dressing is not alkalizing, it adds wonderful flavor when used in moderation on a large plate of fresh greens.

> ¾ cup extra-virgin oil
> ½ cup blueberries (fresh or frozen)
> ⅓ cup cider vinegar
> 6 drops liquid stevia (or to taste)
> Pinch Celtic sea salt or Himalayan salt

1. Place oil, blueberries, vinegar, stevia, and salt in a jar. Cover jar tightly and shake to blend (or use a hand blender).

Tip: Look for cider vinegar with sediment in the bottom, available at most health food stores.

Make ahead: Store in an airtight container in the refrigerator for up to 1 week.

HERB DRESSING

This savory herb dressing is reminiscent of Greek and Italian dressings, and is far more enjoyable than the bottled versions.

> ¾ cup extra-virgin olive oil
> ⅓ cup cider vinegar (see tip, above)
> ½ tsp Celtic sea salt
> 1 tsp dried basil
> ½ tsp dried thyme
> ½ tsp dried oregano
> Pinch cayenne pepper

1. Place oil, vinegar, salt, basil, thyme, oregano, and cayenne in a jar. Cover jar tightly and shake to blend (or use a hand blender).

Make ahead: Store in an airtight container in the refrigerator for up to 2 weeks.

SESAME SENSATION DRESSING   MAKES ABOUT 1 CUP

This dressing can be used over greens or finely chopped vegetables, in place of Caesar salad dressing, or as a dip for crudités. It is packed with alkalizing calcium and fresh lemon juice.

> 1 clove garlic
> Juice of 2 lemons
> ½ cup tahini
> 1 to 2 tbsp organic cold-pressed flaxseed oil
> water

1. In a food processor, process garlic until finely minced. Add lemon juice, tahini, and flaxseed oil; process until smooth. With the motor running, through the feed tube, gradually add water until the desired consistency is achieved (use more water for a salad dressing, less for a dip).

Tip: Tahini, a thick paste made of ground sesame seeds, is available in most health food stores and Lebanese or Middle Eastern markets. Tahini is rich in calcium.

Make ahead: Store in an airtight container in the refrigerator for up to 1 week.

MICHELLE'S QUICK SALAD CROUTONS   MAKES ABOUT 3 CUPS

When you don't have time to make croutons but want some to add to your favorite salad, here's a quick and easy recipe.

> 4 slices sprouted-grain or spelt bread
> 1 to 2 cloves garlic

1. Toast bread until crisp. Rub each slice with garlic and break into bite-sized pieces.

ENTRÉES AND SIDE DISHES

There are many excellent alkalizing meal options. Take time to explore new ways to prepare old favorites, or add some new recipes to your repertoire.

FAJITAS   SERVES 2 TO 4

I could eat these fajitas on a daily basis—they're that good. I'm sure you'll enjoy them too.

  1 tsp dried basil
  ½ tsp ground cumin
  ½ tsp chili powder
  ¼ tsp vegetable salt
  8 oz firm tofu, cut into ½-inch strips
  2 tbsp extra-virgin olive oil
  1 small onion, diced
  1 red bell pepper, diced
  1 large tomato (or 2 small), diced
  1 avocado, diced
  4 sprouted-grain or brown rice tortillas
  Cooked brown rice (see page 172 for cooking instructions)

1. In a small bowl, combine basil, cumin, chili powder, and salt. Add tofu strips and toss to coat.

2. In a skillet, heat 1 tbsp of the oil over medium-low heat, making sure it never smokes. Add seasoned tofu and cook for 3 to 5 minutes per side, or until lightly golden on both sides. Transfer to a plate, cover, and keep warm.

3. In the same skillet, heat the remaining 1 tbsp of olive oil, making sure it never smokes. Sauté onion and red pepper for 10 to 15 minutes, or until onion is golden brown and red pepper has softened.

4. In the center of each tortilla, spoon a line of brown rice, then add tofu, onion, red pepper, tomato, and avocado. Fold in sides of tortilla to hold ingredients together.

RED PEPPER–BUTTERNUT SQUASH QUESADILLAS   Serves 6

Thick puréed butternut squash holds these quesadillas together—and tastes great too!

> 1 tbsp extra-virgin olive oil
> 1 large onion, chopped
> 2 red bell peppers, diced
> 1 package sprouted-grain or brown rice tortillas
> Butternut Squash Tapenade or Roasted Garlic–Butternut Squash
>   Tapenade (see recipes below)
> Vegetable salt

1. In a large skillet, heat oil over medium-low heat, making sure it never smokes. Sauté onion for 5 minutes, or until transparent. Add red peppers and sauté for 10 to 15 minutes, or until peppers are soft and onions are lightly browned.

2. Place one tortilla on each serving plate. Spread tapenade thickly over each tortilla. Spoon onion and red pepper mixture over half of each tortilla. Season with salt to taste. Gently fold tortillas in half and slide into the skillet. Cook, turning once, until warmed through.

BUTTERNUT SQUASH TAPENADE   Makes about 2 cups

> 1 small butternut squash, peeled, seeded, and cubed
> Celtic sea salt or Himalayan salt

1. Place butternut squash in a saucepan. Cover with purified alkaline water and bring to a boil. Reduce heat to low, cover, and simmer for 10 to 15 minutes, or until squash is tender but not mushy. Drain.

2. Transfer to a blender or food processor and purée until smooth (or use a hand blender). Season with salt to taste.

ROASTED GARLIC–BUTTERNUT SQUASH TAPENADE

Prepare Butternut Squash Tapenade (above) and Roasted Garlic Spread (page 153). Add half of the roasted garlic to the tapenade and purée until smooth. (Reserve the remaining roasted garlic for other recipes.)

SLOW COOKER BLACK BEAN CHILI   SERVES 4 TO 6

This yummy black bean chili is perfect for a cold autumn or winter evening, but it's so good you'll probably want to enjoy it in every season.

1½ cups dried black beans
9 cups purified alkaline water, divided
2 tbsp extra-virgin olive oil
2 onions, chopped
3 carrots, chopped
2 red bell peppers, chopped
1 stalk celery, chopped
1 jar (24 oz) tomato sauce
1 cup quinoa
2 tsp ground cumin
1 tsp Celtic sea salt
½ tsp chili powder
Large handful fresh cilantro, chopped

1. In a medium to large slow cooker, combine beans and 6 cups of the water. Cover and cook on low for 6 to 8 hours or overnight, or on high for 3 to 4 hours. Drain and rinse. Return beans to slow cooker.

2. In a large skillet, heat oil over medium-low heat, making sure it never smokes. Sauté onions for 5 minutes. Add carrots, red peppers, and celery; sauté for 10 minutes, or until onions are lightly browned. Transfer to slow cooker.

3. Add tomato sauce, quinoa, cumin, salt, chili powder, cilantro, and the remaining water to the slow cooker. Cover and cook on low for 1 to 1½ hours, or until quinoa is tender.

Tip: Garnish each bowl with a dollop of Avocado Salsa (page 151).

Variation
If you don't have time to slow cook the beans, use 4 cups canned beans, drained and rinsed.

VEGETABLE TAGINE   SERVES 2 TO 4

Don't worry if you don't have an actual Moroccan tagine, a type of cooking dish. You can make this scrumptious one-pot stew without it.

    1 tbsp extra-virgin olive oil
    1 onion, chopped
    1 large carrot (or 2 small), thinly sliced
    1 sweet potato, chopped
    1 stalk celery, chopped
    ½ butternut squash, peeled, seeded, and cubed
    ¼ cup purified alkaline water (approx.)
    1 tsp dried basil
    1 tsp ground cumin
    ½ tsp Celtic sea salt or vegetable salt

1. In a medium saucepan, heat oil over medium-low heat, making sure it never smokes. Sauté onion for 5 minutes. Add carrot and sauté for 5 minutes. Stir in sweet potato, celery, squash, water, basil, cumin, and salt. Cover and simmer, stirring occasionally, for 30 minutes, or until vegetables are tender. Add a small amount of water, if necessary, to prevent sticking.

TUNA-LESS SALAD SANDWICHES   SERVES 2 TO 4

If you love tuna salad sandwiches but want to avoid the mercury and acidity from tuna, you'll love this recipe. This is my favorite use for the fiber- and nutrient-filled pulp left over after juicing carrots. These sandwiches taste great.

    1 stalk celery, finely chopped
    1½ cups carrot pulp (left over from juicing carrots)
    ½ cup finely chopped red or green bell pepper
    2 tbsp minced onion
    ½ tsp Celtic sea salt
    Pinch freshly ground black pepper
    2 tbsp Michelle's Better Butter (see recipe, page 154)
    8 slices sprouted-grain or spelt bread, toasted

1. In a bowl, combine celery, carrot pulp, bell pepper, onion, salt, and pepper. Stir in Michelle's Better Butter until well combined.
2. Spoon vegetable mixture onto 4 slices of toast, pressing down to help the sandwich hold together. Top with the remaining 4 slices of toast.

VEGGIE WRAPS   SERVES 2 TO 4

These wraps make a great meal-on-the go, perfect picnic fare, or a light and easy dinner.

Guacamole or Garlic Guacamole (see recipe, page 152)

2 to 4 sprouted-grain or brown rice tortillas
1 to 2 carrots, shredded
½ cucumber, sliced
½ red and/or green bell pepper, sliced into strips
1 to 2 tomatoes, sliced

1. Spread Guacamole in the center of each tortilla. Place a handful of each vegetable in a line in the center of each tortilla and roll into a wrap.

Variations
Use Hummus (page 152) instead of Guacamole.
Use other raw vegetables of your choice, sliced, chopped, or grated.

HERBED COUSCOUS   SERVES 2 AS AN ENTRÉE OR 4 AS A SIDE DISH

Quinoa, a high-protein ancient grain, stands in for traditional couscous in this fast and easy one-pot dish.

3 tbsp extra-virgin olive oil
1 large onion, chopped
1 small sweet potato, grated
1 stalk celery, finely chopped
2 cups cooked quinoa (see page 172 for cooking instructions)
½ tsp Celtic sea salt
1 tbsp finely chopped fresh basil
1 tbsp finely chopped fresh thyme (leaves only)

1. In a large skillet, heat oil over medium-low heat, making sure it never smokes. Sauté onion for 5 minutes. Add sweet potato and celery; sauté for 10 minutes, or until onion is lightly browned. Add quinoa, salt, basil, and thyme; toss until well combined.

Variation
For a tasty alternative with even more nutrients, add 1 cup diced red bell pepper with the celery.

YAM FRIES   SERVES 2 TO 4

This alternative to french fries tastes better and is far better for you. You can use either yams or sweet potatoes. If you can't tell them apart, yams are a creamy yellow on the inside, while sweet potatoes are a bright salmon-orange color.

    4 yams or sweet potatoes
    2 tbsp extra-virgin olive oil
    1 tsp Celtic sea salt

1. Preheat oven to 350°F. Line a baking sheet with unbleached parchment paper or lightly grease with extra-virgin olive oil or coconut oil.

2. Cut yams into strips similar to french fries. (Try to cut them evenly so they'll cook evenly.) Place in a large bowl, drizzle with oil, and sprinkle with salt. Toss until evenly coated.

3. Place fries in a single layer on prepared baking sheet and bake for 30 minutes. Turn fries over and bake for 30 minutes, or until lightly browned.

DESSERTS

Few desserts are alkalizing. Most sweeteners, whether natural or artificial, are acidifying, as are fruit and chocolate, two common dessert ingredients. But the recipes in this section are healthier options than most. Cinnamon Cookies (page 169) and Chocolate Mousse (page 171) are alkalizing. The other recipes are provided because everyone has a sweet tooth once in a while. Choices that contain natural ingredients and are less acidifying than most packaged or bakery goods will serve your health better over the long term, so you might as well have easy access to them.

BLUEBERRY-STRAWBERRY PUDDING   SERVES 2

You won't believe how easy, delicious, and healthy this pudding is. The acidity of the berries is partially offset by the alkalizing avocado.

   1 avocado, peeled and pitted
   1 container (8 oz) fresh strawberries (or about 10 medium), hulled
   ½ cup frozen blueberries
   30 drops liquid stevia

1. In a food processor, purée avocado, strawberries, blueberries, and stevia until smooth (or use a hand blender). Serve immediately.

CASHEW CREAM   SERVES 2 TO 4

This recipe is acid-forming but is far superior to most desserts, which are both extremely acidic and devoid of nutrition. Cashew Cream is packed with protein and healthy fatty acids. Serve with fresh blueberries, strawberries, or other fruit.

   1 cup unsalted raw cashews
   ½ cup to 1 cup purified alkaline water (depending on desired consistency)
   2 tsp unpasteurized honey

1. In a food processor, finely chop cashews. Add water and honey; purée until creamy.

CINNAMON COOKIES   MAKES ABOUT 24 SMALL COOKIES

Simple and quick to prepare, these cookies are the ideal way to satisfy a sweet tooth, either on their own or with herbal tea.

2 tsp ground psyllium hulls (see tip, page 147)
3 tbsp purified alkaline water
1¼ cup unsalted raw almonds
1 cup old-fashioned oats
½ cup unsweetened, unsalted almond butter
2 tsp ground cinnamon
½ tsp powdered stevia
½ tsp baking soda
Pinch ground ginger
Pinch ground nutmeg

1. Preheat oven to 350ºF and line 2 baking sheets with unbleached parchment paper.

2. In a small bowl, combine psyllium and water; let stand for 5 minutes, until thickened.

3. Meanwhile, in a food processor, grind almonds until fairly fine. Add psyllium mixture, oats, almond butter, cinnamon, stevia, baking soda, ginger, and nutmeg; process until smooth.

4. Shape dough into small, round cookies. Place 2 inches apart on baking sheets and press to ¼-inch thickness. Bake for about 10 minutes, or until lightly golden.

CHOCOLATE CHIP COOKIES   MAKES ABOUT 24 COOKIES

I've included this recipe because chocolate chip cookies are the downfall of many a healthy person, and most store-bought cookies are loaded with white sugar, trans-fat-laden margarine or shortening, preservatives, and many other less-than-healthy ingredients that can push your body well into an acidic condition. These cookies, while still acid-forming, are a better option. That doesn't mean they should be part of your daily diet, or that you should eat more of them. They are meant as an occasional treat only.

2 cups brown rice flour
1½ cups tapioca flour
1 cup organic unrefined sugar
1 tbsp baking powder (see tip below)
3 eggs (approx.)
1 cup extra-virgin coconut oil
2 tsp organic vanilla
1 cup organic dark chocolate chips

1. Preheat oven to 350ºF and line 2 baking sheets with unbleached parchment paper.

2. In a food processor or mixer, combine brown rice flour, tapioca flour, sugar, and baking powder.

3. In a large bowl, beat eggs, oil, and vanilla. Add to dry ingredients and process until dough is soft and slightly shiny. (You may need to add another beaten egg). Stir in chocolate chips.

4. Drop dough by heaping tablespoonfuls 2 inches apart on baking sheets. Bake for 10 to 15 minutes, or until lightly golden.

Tip: Most baking powder contains aluminum, a metal that scientists link with brain disorders such as Alzheimer's disease. Opt for an aluminum-free baking powder, which you can find at your local health food store.

CHOCOLATE MOUSSE   SERVES 2

This is perhaps the world's simplest and healthiest version of chocolate mousse. It can be whipped up in less than 5 minutes. Don't let the ingredient list scare you; you'll be amazed at how good this tastes. It's a wonderful treat for those times when you want something chocolaty. As an added bonus, you'll get lots of usable protein and healthy fatty acids. The avocados are highly alkalizing, which offsets the acidifying effects of the cocoa. And, unlike other desserts, this one won't cause massive blood sugar fluctuations, which are not only hard on the pancreas but zap your energy and make you vulnerable to weight gain. After tasting this decadent treat, you'll understand why it's one of my favorite recipes!

>   2 avocados, peeled and pitted
>   3 tbsp organic unsweetened cocoa powder
>   80 drops liquid stevia (or to taste)

1. In a food processor, purée avocado, cocoa, and stevia until smooth (or use a hand blender). Serve immediately.

COOKING LEGUMES

Rinse dried legumes thoroughly before using, picking out any small stones that have found their way in with the beans. While it is best to soak dried legumes to rehydrate them before cooking, you can skip this step by cooking them in a slow cooker on low. I start them cooking at night before I go to bed. When I awaken, the beans are ready to be rinsed and added to recipes. If you're cooking legumes on the stovetop, you'll need to soak them for at least 1 hour, and preferably overnight. For every cup of dried beans, add 4 cups of purified alkaline water. Discard the soaking water to reduce the gas-forming potential of the beans. Cook each cup of legumes in 4 cups of fresh water, bringing the water to a boil and then reducing the heat to low and simmering until legumes are tender but not mushy. Depending on the type of bean, cooking usually takes between 30 and 90 minutes.

COOKING WHOLE GRAINS

In a pot, combine grain and purified alkaline water (see chart, below, for amounts). Add a drizzle of olive oil, if desired, and a pinch of Celtic sea salt. Cover and bring to a boil. Reduce heat to low and simmer for the cooking time indicated on chart below. Whole grains can be served on their own or used as a base for steamed or stir-fried vegetables. You can also add Almond Milk (page 145) to cooked grains such as millet or quinoa, along with stevia to taste, and heat for a delectable hot breakfast cereal or pudding.

COOKING CHART FOR WISE ACID AND ALKALINE WHOLE GRAINS

Grain	Acid- or Alkaline- Forming	Amount of Grain	Amount of Water	Cooking Time	Yield (approximate)
Oats, quick-cooking	Moderately acidic	1 cup	3 cups	12 to 20 minutes	2½ cups
Oats, old-fashioned	Moderately acidic	1 cup	2 to 3 cups	40 to 50 minutes	4 cups
Brown rice	Moderately acidic	1 cup	2 cups	35 to 40 minutes	2½ cups
Wild rice	Moderately acidic	1 cup	3 cups	50 to 60 minutes	3 to 4 cups
Amaranth	Slightly acidic	1 cup	2 cups	25 to 30 minutes	2½ cups
Kasha	Slightly acidic	1 cup	1¾ cups	15 to 20 minutes	2½ cups
Millet	Slightly acidic	1 cup	2½ cups	30 minutes	4 cups
Triticale	Slightly acidic	1 cup	3 cups	60 minutes	3½ cups
Buckwheat groats	Slightly alkaline	1 cup	2 cups	15 minutes	2 to 2½ cups
		1 cup	2 cups	20 minutes	2¾ cups
		1 cup	2½ cups	45 to 60 minutes	3 cups

Acknowledgments

In my life, I am surrounded by wonderful, caring people of integrity and compassion who support me in my work and personal life. I would like to extend my thanks to everyone who contributed to this book and offered their wisdom, guidance, and support throughout the research, writing, and editing processes.

To my soulmate and life partner, Curtis: Thank you for your unending love and support . . . always. You are undoubtedly an earth angel. This book could not have happened without your constant support, your selfless and immense assistance, and your patience throughout this project. I am blessed to share life with you. You are truly the kindest, wisest, and most caring man I've ever met. I know love because I know you. I thank the heavens for the day you walked into my life—November 21, 1997—the second-happiest day of my life, second only to the day we exchanged our wedding vows. You have changed my life more than you will ever know. Whatever our souls are made of, yours and mine are the same. Thank you, my beautiful love.

To Claire Gerus, my wonderful agent: Thanks for suggesting that I write this book and for your tremendous assistance with its development. Thanks also for your wisdom, kindness, support, and friendship.

To Harvey Diamond: Thanks for writing the foreword for this book. Your life and work are an inspiration to millions of people—including me. I am honored to have your support. Your kindness and generosity of spirit are immensely appreciated.

To Rick Broadhead: Thanks for your help in finding a good home for this book.

To Brad and Anne at HarperCollins: Thank you for the many hours you spent turning my manuscript into a book that I am proud of.

To Noelle: Thanks for your excellent work managing this book process. It was a pleasure working with you.

To Sue Sumeraj: Thanks for the expert copyediting and for sharing your delicious juice recipe.

To Mom and Dad: You are wonderful, loving parents whose friendship and encouragement I value immensely. I cherish you, your faith in me, and your love and support.

To Bob: Thanks for the great recipes you shared, for your friendship, and for the laughs—you always make me laugh. You're a great sister.

To Juniper: You really outdid yourself! Thanks.

To Father Ron: Thanks for always watching out for me and for guiding and inspiring me, even on the other side.

To everyone else at HarperCollins who contributed to this book: Thank you.

Thank you to all my wonderful and supportive friends.

In everyone's life, a teacher stands out as someone who sees our potential and guides us to fulfill it. Thank you, Mr. Paul McInnes, for your words of wisdom and your kindness, and for seeing and guiding my potential.

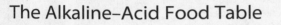

The Alkaline–Acid Food Table

The table below shows common foods ranging from alkaline to acidic. Eating foods from the left side of the chart will help you maintain your body's pH in a healthy range. If you eat food from the right side of the chart—and most people do—simply remember to minimize the frequency and the portion, and supplement with greater amounts of alkaline foods.

Food Type	Most Alkaline	Moderately Alkaline	Slightly Alkaline	Slightly Acidic	Moderately Acidic	Most Acidic
Dairy Products and Milk Alternatives	Human breast milk		Goat's milk	Cow's milk Cream Rice milk Soy milk		Cheese (milk, goat, soy) Ice cream Yogurt Whey Casein
Meat, Poultry, and Fish				Fish, wild, freshwater	Fish, wild, ocean	Beef Veal Pork Organ meats Poultry Eggs Shellfish Fish, farmed
Vegetables	Cucumbers Dandelion greens Kale Sea vegetables (such as agar, arame, dulse, hijiki, and nori) Sprouted beans (including soy sprouts)	Arugula Beets Broccoli Cabbage Celery Collard greens Endive Garlic Gingerroot Green beans Mustard greens Okra Onions	Artichokes Asparagus Brussels sprouts Carrots Cauliflower Chives Horseradish Kohlrabi Leeks Peas Rhubarb Rutabaga Sweet potatoes			Potatoes (white or red)

Food Type	Most Alkaline	Moderately Alkaline	Slightly Alkaline	Slightly Acidic	Moderately Acidic	Most Acidic
Vegetables	Sprouted seeds (e.g., alfalfa, red clover, and broccoli)	Peppers, bell Peppers, hot (fresh, not pickled) Radishes Salad greens Sorrel Spinach	Turnips Watercress Yams Zucchini			
Legumes	Soy lecithin and soy nuts	Edamame (green soybeans) Lima beans Navy beans	Lentils Soy flour Tofu	Black beans Chickpeas Kidney beans		
Fruit		Avocados	Cherries (sour) Coconut Grapefruit Lemons Limes Tomatoes	Cantaloupe Dates (fresh) Nectarines Plums	Apples Apricots Bananas Berries Cherries (sweet) Currants Figs (fresh) Grapes Guava Honeydew melon Mangos Oranges Papayas Peaches Pears Persimmons Pineapple Tangerines Watermelon	All dried, pickled, or canned fruit
Grains			Buckwheat groats or flour Quinoa Spelt grains or flour Spelt bread (yeast-free, sugar-free and preservative-free)	Amaranth Kasha Millet Triticale	Brown rice Wild rice Oats Rye bread White bread Whole-grain bread	Barley (pearl or pot) Corn Oat bran

Food Type	Most Alkaline	Moderately Alkaline	Slightly Alkaline	Slightly Acidic	Moderately Acidic	Most Acidic
Nuts and Seeds	Pumpkin seeds		Almonds (raw, unsalted) Caraway seeds Cumin seeds Fennel seeds Sesame seeds	Brazil nuts Hazelnuts Pecans Flaxseeds Sunflower seeds	Walnuts	Cashews Peanuts Pistachios
Herbs and Spices	Celtic sea salt Himalayan salt	Fresh and dried herbs: basil, cilantro, oregano, parsley, rosemary, sage, thyme, etc. Cayenne pepper		Curry powder	Nutmeg Table salt Vanilla	
Condiments and Extras					Ketchup Mayonnaise	Carob Cocoa Jam/jelly Malt MSG Mustard Rice syrup Soy sauce Vinegar
Oils and Fats			Almond oil Avocado oil Borage oil Coconut oil Cod liver oil Evening primrose oil Flaxseed oil Olive oil Soy oil	Canola oil Grapeseed oil Sunflower oil Walnut oil	Butter Corn oil Margarine	

Food Type	Most Alkaline	Moderately Alkaline	Slightly Alkaline	Slightly Acidic	Moderately Acidic	Most Acidic
Sweeteners			Chicory Stevia			Agave nectar All artificial sweeteners and sugar substitutes Beet sugar Corn syrup Honey (pasteurized and un-pasteurized) Molasses White sugar
Beverages	Alkaline water Fresh vegetable juice		Distilled water		Fruit juice, natural un-processed	Alcohol (including beer and wine) Coffee Fruit juice, processed and sweetened Tea Soft drinks Sports drinks

Clearly, a meal of steak, french fries (with salt, vinegar, and ketchup), a beer or cola, and chocolate cake can throw your whole system off. Add a cup of coffee and you're quickly running a serious alkaline mineral deficit. Once your addictive cravings are gone and your body has detoxified from acid-forming foods and acid wastes, you will find yourself craving the delicious alkaline foods that fuel your body and provide energy.

The Facts about Water Filtration

It can be difficult to find alkaline water from traditional sources, let alone water that will have a significant alkalizing effect on our body. And yet alkaline water gives us tremendous health benefits. Remember how much water is required to neutralize the acidity from one glass of cola? No one can drink that much water, so the alternative is to create water that is more alkaline than the liquid found in our taps or bottles. There are a couple of ways to do that, but let's discuss filtration first.

The quest for pure, alkaline water has led to considerable growth in the water filtration industry—and considerable growth in unscrupulous products, gimmicks, and schemes as well. No filter will remove every contaminant. Specific filtration technologies tend to focus on a certain type of water problem. Some are better at removing inorganic pollutants, such as heavy metals and chemicals, while others are more effective on organic intruders, such as viruses and bacteria. Generally, you get what you pay for. For example, those clear plastic jugs with replaceable filters are not doing a whole lot of filtering. They are better than nothing until they get older and become "polluted" as well—which happens quite quickly—and then bacteria start to grow in the carbon filters. You need to stay on top of them and change the filters regularly. And their ability to make your water less acidic is negligible.

It is important to do your homework to find the best option for your water needs. Many water filtration and/or purification systems combine different filter technologies to eliminate or reduce pollutants. Here are some of the more common types:[1]

Activated carbon: A pound of carbon has a surface area of 125 acres and can absorb thousands of different contaminants. It is particularly effective on bad tastes and odors, chlorine, radon, most sediment, and volatile organic compounds (VOCs), but has little ability to alkalize water. Activated carbon filtration systems are available in many forms, including under-the-counter and counter-top options and units that fit inside pitchers and even in personal water bottles.

KDF-55: This filtration option is a copper–zinc formula that relies on a chemical process called oxidation/reduction (redox) to remove pollutants from the water. It is effective on bad tastes and odors, heavy metals, chlorine, hydrogen sulfide, and iron but has little ability to alkalize water.

Reverse osmosis: This hyper-filtration method uses both pre-filters (such as activated carbon) and membranes with unbelievably small pores to trap contaminants. As such, it is effective for bacteria and viruses, arsenic, fluoride, nitrates, and most of the substances identified above. It is moderately effective on VOCs and hydrogen sulfide and ineffective on radon.

Ultraviolet (UV) light: UV light is a form of radiation, effective at killing pathogens such as viruses, molds, algae, bacteria, and yeasts. It has proven effective against cryptosporidium and giardia. UV filtration's Achilles heel is chemicals and heavy metals, so to be truly effective it is best combined with another filtration process.

Distilled water: Distilled water is a controversial topic in the natural health field. Distilled water is, for all intents and purposes, hydrogen and oxygen. There are no added minerals, and those that existed prior to distillation are removed. The strongest claims against distilled water, which have persisted for years, suggest that it is devoid of minerals and actually leaches minerals out of your body, damaging your teeth and bones. We get most of our minerals from a healthy diet of fruits, vegetables, and whole grains. Water is a minor source of minerals. Distilled water does not leach minerals from your body—this false claim is typically made by people selling a competing type of water purification system. The only minerals that distilled water affects are those that have been used or are not useable by the body and need to be eliminated, such as toxic metals. Distilled water helps the blood escort these wastes out of the body.

Distillation helps eliminate or reduce both organic and inorganic compounds in water. It also has a pH around 7.0, which would be great if it was the only thing you drank and your diet was already alkaline. Unfortunately, the Standard American Diet is extremely acidic; to help fight the acidity, you need water with a higher pH. Distilled water is a healthy option alongside a highly alkaline diet, but it cannot counter the effects of an acidic diet.

Ionized water: Without getting too scientific, an ion is an atom with a positive or negative charge. Our bodies are electric systems—every cell has a charge. An acidic state produces a great many positive ions, which on closer examination are not so positive. Many toxins, chemicals, noxious gases, and other pollutants in our food and air enter our bodies as positive ions. We need negative ions to bind with them (opposites attract) and neutralize them. Otherwise, carbon dioxide and other acidic wastes build up in the body.

Water ionizers use an electrolysis or ionization process to alter water molecules to form both negatively charged and positively charged water. The former is alkaline water, which helps our bodies function and eliminate acidic waste. The latter is acidic water, which can be used for other non-life-sustaining purposes, such as housecleaning. Through the ionization process, the water is also altered at the molecular level, rendering it more useable and allowing the drinker to hydrate more quickly.

Ionized water's benefits for human health have been studied more meticulously in Asia than in North America. Studies from Japan and Korea have illustrated links between alkaline ionized water and lower blood sugar levels in diabetics, improved liver function, reduced allergy symptoms, and decreased acid levels in people with gout.[2] You may recall that high acidity has been linked to all of these conditions.

I strongly encourage you to invest in an alkalizing water filtration system. Yes, they can be pricy, but an alkalizing water filtration system may be one of the best investments you can make for your health. If you can't afford one, or you want to further increase the alkalizing power of your water, simply add baking soda, fresh lemon juice, or alkalizing drops to pure water.

Resources

CELLFOOD®

Cellfood is a unique cell-oxygenating liquid formula that delivers 78 trace minerals, 34 enzymes, 17 amino acids, and electrolytes and increases the bioavailability of oxygen to the body using a unique water-splitting technology. It is readily absorbed by the body at the cellular level, making a wealth of nutrients available to your cells for optimum healing. Unlike other products I've tried, Cellfood delivers the oxygen slowly, thereby preventing free radical damage. Cellfood also helps normalize an acidic pH (which is integral to proper detoxification and healing), assists with energy, and boosts the immune system. I recommend adding eight drops of Cellfood to a glass of pure water or juice three times per day.

Cellfood is available at most health food stores and from health care practitioners. For more information, contact Lumina Health Products at www.luminahealth.com or 1-800-749-9196, or by sending an email to info@luminahealth.com.

EXERCISE VIDEO

Pain Free Mobility Exercises is an exercise DVD that I find quite helpful. It teaches a great series of exercises that encourage flexibility and lessen pain. I've tried many other exercise videos, but this one is different—it can be done by exercise novices and athletes alike, and is also suitable for people recovering from injuries or with other physical limitations. Developed by two registered massage therapists with a strong knowledge of the body, *Pain Free Mobility Exercises* can be done in just 15 minutes a day, but you'll feel lasting benefits. For more information, visit www.advancedbowentherapy.com.

JUICERS

Whether you buy a $40 juicer or a $400 juicer, you are doing your body a huge favor by juicing every day. Most of the popular kitchen equipment manufacturers offer juicers at reasonable prices. These models often use a spinning technique that, according to some experts, introduces a great deal of air into the juice, leading it to oxidize faster, which means the nutrients lose their value more quickly. The more expensive juicers use a mastication, or chewing, process to break down the fibers and cellular material in vegetables and fruit, giving you more useable fiber, enzymes, vitamins, and trace minerals, all of which enhance the health benefits of your juice. These juicers are heavy-duty, multi-purpose machines and can also be used to make baby food, fresh nut butters, and healthy frozen desserts. I use a Champion juicer for standard juicing, and I also like the Green Star juicer. To make whole juices, I use a Vita-Mix high-powered blender.

SOY MILK MAKERS

Soy milk is a great substitute for dairy milk and offers numerous health benefits. Store brands, however, often contain sugar and other additives. Soy milk makers allow you to make additive-free milk from fresh water and soybeans. You combine the ingredients, and the machine does the rest. Homemade soy milk isn't for everyone—it's an acquired taste. I enjoy it best as an ingredient in a smoothie or a dish I am making.

There are a number of different brands of soy milk makers, such as Soy Quick (formerly Soy Life) and SoyJoy. For additional information, check out www.soymilkmaker.com or www.soymilkquick.com.

SUPER SIZE ME

If you want to see how quickly a highly acidic diet can mess with your health, I urge you to buy or rent the award-winning film *Super Size Me*. It is shocking, amusing, and sad all at the same time. Filmmaker Morgan Spurlock spent a month eating nothing but fast food from McDonald's—morning, noon, and night—and traveled across the United States, interviewing fast-food fanatics, health experts, lawyers, industry association mouthpieces, and kids about the fast-food debate.

VITA-MIX BLENDER/TOTAL JUICER

The Vita-Mix is not your standard blender. While it is a bit costly (currently between $400 and $600), it is worth every penny. I have had my Vita-Mix for eight years, and a rare day goes by that I don't use it at least once. I use it to make smoothies, whole juices, and even soups. It also comes with a dry blade canister for grinding grains. To learn more about the Vita-Mix blender, visit www.vitamix.com.

Notes

CHAPTER 1: The Fatal Flaws in Our Standard American Diet (SAD)

[1] Schoffro Cook, *Brain Wash*, 82.
[2] Mittelstaedt, "'Inherently Toxic.'"
[3] Ibid.
[4] Melcombe, *Health Hazards*, 30.
[5] Tephly and McMartin, "Methanol Metabolism."
[6] Kristensen et al., "Short-Term Effects"; Johnson, "Multifaceted and Widespread Pathology."
[7] Tucker et al., "Colas, But Not Other Carbonated Beverages"; Wykshak and Frisch, "Carbonated Beverages."
[8] Manz, "History of Nutrition."
[9] Sebastian et al., "Estimation of the Net Acid Load."
[10] Krop, *Healing the Planet*, 75.

CHAPTER 2: Maintaining a Delicate Balance

[1] Environment Canada, "Acid Rain."
[2] Kalhoff and Manz. "Nutrition, Acid-Base Status."
[3] Boyle, "Lymphatic Stress."
[4] Dancey, *Cellulite Solution*.
[5] Bushinsky, "Acid-Base Imbalance."

CHAPTER 3: The Acid–Disease Connection

[1] Frasetto et al., "Diet, Evolution."
[2] Clarke et al., "Folate, Vitamin B_{12}."
[3] Pirchl, Marksteiner, and Humpel, "Effects of Acidosis."
[4] Panush et al., "Food-Induced ('Allergic') Arthritis."
[5] Levy et al., "Dietary Fat."
[6] Kjeldsen-Kragh et al., "Controlled Trial."
[7] Schoffro Cook, *Healing Injuries*, 23.
[8] Bushinsky, "Acid-Base Imbalance."
[9] As cited in Graci, DeMarco, and Rao, *Bone-Building Solution*, 178.
[10] Young and Young, *Sick and Tired*, 36.
[11] Singh, "Mitochondrial Dysfunction."
[12] Smallbone et al., "Metabolic Changes."
[13] Koukourakis et al., "Oxygen and Glucose Consumption."
[14] Ihnatko et al., "Extracellular Acidosis."
[15] Racciatti et al., "Chronic Fatigue Syndrome."
[16] Lipscombe, "Targeting High-Risk Populations."
[17] Cameron et al., "Urine Composition."

[18] Young and Young, *The pH Miracle for Diabetes.*
[19] As cited at http://whale.to/v/disease3.html.
[20] Young and Young, *The pH Miracle for Weight Loss.*
[21] Kraut and Kurtz, "Metabolic Acidosis of CKD"; Klahr and Morrissey, "Progression of Chronic Renal Disease"; Bailey, "Metabolic Acidosis."
[22] Graci, DeMarco, and Rao, *Bone-Building Solution.*
[23] Karagülle et al., "Clinical Study."
[24] Tamarro, McGarry, and Cyr, "Perioperative Care."
[25] Lesch Kelly, "Dairy Debate."
[26] Harvey Diamond, unpublished interview with Michelle Schoffro Cook, April 2004.
[27] As quoted in Lesch Kelly, "Dairy Debate."
[28] Manson, "Nurses' Health Study."
[29] Willett, "Health Professionals."
[30] As quoted in Lesch Kelly, "Dairy Debate."
[31] Ibid.
[32] Frassetto et al., "Estimation of Net."
[33] Tucker et al., "Colas, But Not Other Carbonated Beverages."
[34] Kristensen et al., "Short-Term Effects."
[35] McKenzie, "Study: Depression."
[36] Graci, DeMarco, and Rao, *Bone-Building Solution*, 181.
[37] Maurer et al., "Neutralization of Western Diet."
[38] Young and Young, *Sick and Tired*, 49.

CHAPTER 4: Making Wise Acid Choices

[1] Appleton, *Lick the Sugar Habit*, 11.
[2] Galli et al., "Blueberry Supplemented Diet."
[3] Joseph et al., "Reversals of Age-Related Declines."
[4] Mercola, "Keep Alzheimer's Away."
[5] Young and Young, *Sick and Tired*, 71.
[6] Ibid., 72.

CHAPTER 5: Alkalizing for Lasting Health

[1] Goodfriend, "Better Than Red Wine."
[2] Young and Young, *The pH Miracle for Weight Loss*, 65–68.
[3] Ibid., 60.

CHAPTER 6: Choosing the Best Alkaline-Friendly Supplements

[1] Ong et al., "Chlorophyllin."
[2] Mercola, "Chlorella."
[3] Barth, Guseo, and Klein, "In Vitro Study."
[4] Jehle et al., "Partial Neutralization."
[5] Institute of Medicine, *Dietary Reference Intakes*, 8.

CHAPTER 7: The Kick Acid Lifestyle

[1] For more information on tai chi and the National Institutes of Health's National Center for Complementary and Alternative Medicine's research on tai chi, visit http://nccam.nih.gov/health/taichi.

[2]   Sha, *Power Healing*, 77.

[3]   Ibid., 79–80.

[4]   Barnes et al., *Complementary and Alternative Medicine*.

[5]   For more information on meditation and the National Institutes of Health's National Center for Complementary and Alternative Medicine's research on meditation, visit: http://nccam.nih.gov/health/meditation.

[6]   As quoted in Kusek Lewis, "Massage."

[7]   For more information on acupuncture and the National Institute of Health's National Center for Complementary and Alternative Medicine's research on acupuncture, visit: http://nccam.nih.gov/health/acupuncture.

[8]   National Center for Complementary and Alternative Medicine, "Acupuncture for Osteoarthritis."

[9]   de Vernejoul, Albarède, and Darras, "Study of Acupuncture."

[10]   Benor, *Spiritual Healing*.

[11]   Barak, "Immune System."

[12]   Kubzansky et al., "Is the Glass Half Empty?"

[13]   Kubzansky et al., "Is Worrying Bad?"

APPENDIX B: The Facts about Water Filtration

[1]   To learn more about water purification options, visit www.home-water-purifiers-and-filters.com.

[2]   For a summary of the results of these studies, visit www.lifeionizers.com.

Bibliography

Appleton, Nancy. *Lick the Sugar Habit*. New York: Avery, 1996.

Bailey, J.L. "Metabolic Acidosis: An Unrecognized Cause of Morbidity in the Patient with Chronic Kidney Disease." *Kidney International* 96, Supplement (July 2005): S15–23.

Barak, Yoram. "The Immune System and Happiness." *Autoimmunity Reviews* 5, no. 8 (October 2006): 523–27.

Barnes, P., E. Powell-Griner, K. McFann, and R. Nahin. *Complementary and Alternative Medicine Use among Adults: United States, 2002*. Advance Data Report #343. Natural Standard, May 27, 2004.

Barth, H., A. Guseo, and R. Klein. "In Vitro Study on the Immunological Effects of Bromelain and Trypsin on Mononuclear Cells from Humans." *European Journal of Medical Research* 10, no. 8 (2005): 325–31.

Benor, Daniel J. *Spiritual Healing: Scientific Validation of a Healing Revolution*. Southfield, MI: Vision Publications, 2001.

Boyle, Jillian. "Is Lymphatic Stress the Reason You're Fat? Bloated? Hungry for Junk Food?" *Woman's World*, March 2, 2004.

Bushinsky, David A. "Acid-Base Imbalance and the Skeleton." *European Journal of Nutrition* 40, no. 5 (October 2001): 238–44.

Cameron, M.A., N.M. Maalouf, B. Adams-Huet, O.W. Moe, and K. Sakhaee. "Urine Composition in Type 2 Diabetes: Predisposition to Uric Acid Nephrolithiasis." *Journal of the American Society of Nephrology* 17, no. 5 (May 2006): 1422–28.

Campbell, T. Colin, with Thomas M. Campbell II. *The China Study: Startling Implications for Diet, Weight Loss and Long-Term Health*. Dallas: BenBella Books, 2005.

Clarke, R., A.D. Smith, K.A. Jobst, H. Refsum, L. Sutton, and P.M. Ueland. "Folate, Vitamin B_{12}, and Serum Total Homocysteine Levels in Confirmed Alzheimer Disease." *Archives of Neurology* 55, no. 11 (November 1998): 1449–55.

Dancey, Elisabeth. *The Cellulite Solution*. Philadelphia: Coronet, 1996.

de Vernejoul, P., P. Albarède, and J.C. Darras. "Study of Acupuncture Meridians Using Radioactive Tracers." *Bulletin de l'Académie Nationale de Médecine* 169, no. 7 (October 1985): 1071–75.

Environment Canada. "Acid Rain and . . . Forests." May 19, 2005. Available at: www.ec.gc.ca/acidrain/acidforest.html.

Fleming, R.M. "The Effects of High-Protein Diets on Coronary Blood Flow." *Angiology* 51, no. 10 (October 2000): 817–26.

Frassetto, L., R.C. Morris, D.E. Sellmeyer, K. Todd, and A. Sebastian. "Diet, Evolution and Aging: The Pathophysiologic Effects of the Post-Agricultural Inversion of the Potassium-to-Sodium and Base-to-Chloride Ratios in the Human Diet." *European Journal of Nutrition* 40, no. 5 (October 2001): 200–213.

Frassetto, L.A., K.M. Todd, R.C. Morris, and A. Sebastian. "Estimation of Net Endogenous Noncarbonic Acid Production in Humans from Diet Potassium and Protein Contents." *American Journal of Clinical Nutrition* 68, no. 3 (September 1998): 576–83.

Galli, R.L., D.F. Bielinski, A. Szprengiel, B. Shukitt-Hale, and J.A. Joseph. "Blueberry Supplemented Diet Reverses Age-Related Decline in Hippocampal HSP70 Neuroprotection." *Neurobiological Aging* 27, no. 2 (February 2006): 344–50.

Goodfriend, Anne "Better Than Red Wine or Green Tea?" *USA Today*, March 2, 2006. Available at: www.usatoday.com/travel/destinations/2006-03-02-yerba-benefits_x.htm.

Graci, Sam, Carolyn DeMarco, and Leticia Rao. *The Bone-Building Solution*. Toronto: John Wiley & Sons, 2006.

Ihnatko, R., M. Kubes, M. Takacova, O. Sedlakova, J. Sedlak, J. Pastorek, J. Kopacek, and S. Pastorekova. "Extracellular Acidosis Elevates Carbonic Anhydrase IX in Human Glioblastoma Cells via Transcriptional Modulation That Does Not Depend on Hypoxia." *International Journal of Oncology* 29, no. 4 (October 2006): 1025–33.

Institute of Medicine. *Dietary Reference Intakes for Thiamin, Riboflavin, Niacin, Vitamin B_6, Folate, Vitamin B_{12}, Pantothenic Acid, Biotin, and Choline*. Washington, DC: National Academy Press, 2000.

Jehle, S., A. Zanetti, J. Muser, H.N. Hulter, and R. Krapf. "Partial Neutralization of the Acidogenic Western Diet with Potassium Citrate Increases Bone Mass in Postmenopausal Women with Osteopenia." *Journal of the American Society of Nephrology* 17, no. 11 (November 2006): 3213–22.

Johnson, S. "The Multifaceted and Widespread Pathology of Magnesium Deficiency." *Medical Hypotheses* 56, no. 2 (February 2001):163-70.

Joseph, J.A., B. Shukitt-Hale, N.A. Denisova, D. Bielinski, A. Martin, J.J. McEwen, and P.C. Bickford. "Reversals of Age-Related Declines in Neuronal Signal Transduction, Cognitive, and Motor Behavioral Deficits with Blueberry, Spinach, or Strawberry Dietary Supplementation." *Journal of Neuroscience* 19, no. 18 (September 15, 1999): 8114–21.

Kalhoff, Hermann, and Freidrich Manz. "Nutrition, Acid-Base Status and Growth in Early Childhood." *European Journal of Nutrition* 40, no. 5 (October 2001): 221–30.

Karagülle, O., U. Smorag, F. Candir, G. Gundermann, U. Jonas, A.J. Becker, A. Gehrke, and C. Gutenbrunner. "Clinical Study on the Effect of Mineral Waters Containing Bicarbonate on the Risk of Urinary Stone Formation in Patients with Multiple Episodes of CaOx-Urolithiasis." *World Journal of Urology* 25, no. 3 (June 2007): 315–23.

Kjeldsen-Kragh, J., M. Haugen, C.F. Borchgrevink, E. Laerum, M. Eek, P. Mowinkel, K. Hovi, and O. Forre. "Controlled Trial of Fasting and One-Year Vegetarian Diet in Rheumatoid Arthritis." *The Lancet* 338, no. 8772 (October 12, 1991): 899–902.

Klahr, S., and J. Morrissey. "Progression of Chronic Renal Disease." *American Journal of Kidney Disease* 41, no. 3, Supplement 1 (March 2003): S3–7.

Koukourakis, M.I., M. Pitiakoudis, A. Giatromanolaki, A. Tsarouha, A. Polychronidis, E. Sivridis, and C. Simopoulos. "Oxygen and Glucose Consumption in Gastrointestinal Adenocarcinomas: Correlation with Markers of Hypoxia, Acidity and Anaerobic Glycolysis." *Cancer Science* 97, no. 10 (October 2006): 1056–60.

Kraut, J.A., and I. Kurtz. "Metabolic Acidosis of CKD: Diagnosis, Clinical Characteristics, and Treatment." *American Journal of Kidney Disease* 45, no. 6 (June 2005): 978–93.

Kristensen, M., M. Jensen, J. Kudsk, M. Henriksen, and C. Molgaard. "Short-Term Effects on Bone Turnover of Replacing Milk with Cola Beverages: A 10-Day Interventional Study in Young Men." *Osteoporosis International* 16, no. 12 (December 2005): 1803–8.

Krop, Jozef J. *Healing the Planet One Patient at a Time.* Caledon: KOS, 2002.

Kubzansky, L.D., I. Kawachi, A. Spiro, S.T. Weiss, P.S. Vokonas, and D. Sparrow. "Is Worrying Bad for Your Heart? A Prospective Study of Worry and Coronary Heart Disease in the Normative Aging Study." *Circulation* 95, no. 4 (February 18, 1997): 818–24.

Kubzansky L.D., D. Sparrow, P. Vokonas, and I. Kawachi. "Is the Glass Half Empty or Half Full? A Prospective Study of Optimism and Coronary Heart Disease in the Normative Aging Study." *Psychosomatic Medicine* 63, no. 6 (November–December 2001): 910–16.

Kusek Lewis, Krysten. "Massage: It's Real Medicine." *Health,* February 2007. Available at: http://www.health.com/health/article/0,23414,1591705,00.html.

Lesch Kelly, Alice. "The Dairy Debate: Does Milk Build Stronger Bones?" *Los Angeles Times,* March 7, 2005. Available at: www.thechinastudy.com/la-times-article.html.

Levy, J.A., A.B. Ibrahim, T. Shirai, K. Ohta, R. Nagasawa, H. Yoshida, J. Estes, and M. Gardner. "Dietary Fat Affects Immune Response, Production of Antiviral Factors, and Immune Complex Disease in NZP/NZW Mice." *Proceedings of the National Academy of Sciences* 79, no. 6 (March 1982): 1974–78.

Lipscombe, Lorraine. "Targeting High-Risk Populations in the Fight Against Diabetes." *The Lancet* 369, no. 9563 (March 3, 2007): 716.

Manson, Joanne. "Nurses' Health Study." August 1, 2007. Available at: http://clinicaltrials.gov/show/NCT00005152.

Manz, Freidrich. "History of Nutrition and Acid-Base Physiology." *European Journal of Nutrition* 40, no. 5 (October 2001): 189–99.

Maurer, M., W. Riesen, J. Muser, H. Hulter, and R. Krapf. "Neutralization of Western Diet Inhibits Bone Resorption Independently of K Intake and Reduces Cortisol Secretion in Humans." *American Journal of Physiology – Renal Physiology* 284, no. 1 (January 2003): F32–40.

McKenzie, John. "Study: Depression Causes Brittle Bones." *ABC News*, January 13, 2007. Available at: http://abcnews.go.com/WNT/Depression/story?id=129893.

Melcombe, Lynne. *Health Hazards of White Sugar.* Vancouver: Alive Books, 2001.

Mercola, Joseph. "Chlorella: A Natural Wonder Food." 2005. Available at: http://cmsadmin.mercola.com/chlorella/index.htm.

———. "Keep Alzheimer's Away with Fish Oil's Secret Weapon." April 6, 2005. Available at: www.mercola.com/2005/apr/6/alzheimers_fish_oil.htm.

Mittelstaedt, Martin. "'Inherently Toxic' Chemical Faces Its Future." *The Globe and Mail*, April 8, 2007.

Murray, Michael. "Good Health and Optimism Go Hand in Hand." *Health & Wellness Newsletter* (Spring 2004).

National Center for Complementary and Alternative Medicine. National Institutes of Health. "Acupuncture for Osteoarthritis of the Knee Study Results." December 20, 2004. Available at: http://nccam.nih.gov/research/results/acu-osteo.htm.

Ong, T.M., W.Z. Whong, J. Stewart, and H.E. Brockman. "Chlorophyllin: A Potent Antimutagen Against Environmental and Dietary Complex Mixtures." *Mutational Research* 173, no. 2 (February 1986): 111–15.

Panush, R.S. "Food-Induced ('Allergic') Arthritis: Clinical and Serologic Studies." *Journal of Rheumatology* 17, no. 3 (March 1990): 291–94.

Panush R.S., E.M. Webster, L.P. Endo, J.M. Greer, and J.C. Woodard. "Food-Induced ("Allergic") Arthritis: Inflammatory Synovitis in Rabbits." *Journal of Rheumatology.* 17, no. 3 (March 1990): 285–90.

Pirchl, M., J. Marksteiner, and C. Humpel. "Effects of Acidosis on Brain Capillary Endothelial Cells and Cholinergic Neurons: Relevance to Vascular Dementia and Alzheimer's Disease." *Neurological Research* 28, no. 6 (September 2006): 657–64.

Racciatti, D., J. Vecchiet, A. Ceccomancini, F. Ricci, and E. Pizzigallo. "Chronic Fatigue Syndrome Following a Toxic Exposure." *The Science of the Total Environment* 270, nos. 1–3 (April 10, 2001): 27–31.

Root, Leon. *Beautiful Bones Without Hormones: The All-New Natural Diet and Exercise Program to Reduce the Risk of Osteoporosis.* New York: Gotham Books, 2004.

Schoffro Cook, Michelle. *The Brain Wash: A Powerful, All-Natural Program to Protect Your Brain Against Alzheimer's, Chronic Fatigue Syndrome, Depression, Parkinson's and Other Diseases.* Toronto: John Wiley & Sons, 2007.

————. *Healing Injuries the Natural Way: How to Mend Bones, Muscles, Tendons, and More.* Toronto: Your Health Press, 2004.

Sebastian, A., L.A. Frassetto, D.E. Sellmeyer, R.L. Merriam, and C. Morris, Jr. "Estimation of the Net Acid Load of the Diet of Ancestral Preagricultural *Homo Sapiens* and Their Hominid Ancestors." *American Journal of Clinical Nutrition* 76, no. 6 (December 2002): 803–4.

Sha, Zhi Gang. *Power Healing: The Four Keys to Energizing Your Body, Mind and Spirit.* New York: HarperCollins, 2002.

Singh, K.K. "Mitochondrial Dysfunction Is a Common Phenotype in Aging and Cancer." *Annals of the New York Academy of Sciences* 1019 (June 2004): 260–64.

Smallbone, K., R.A. Gatenby, R.J. Gillies, P.K. Maini, and D.J. Gavaghan. "Metabolic Changes During Carcinogenesis: Potential Impact on Invasiveness." *Journal of Theoretical Biology* 244, no. 4 (February 21, 2007): 703–13.

Tamarro, D., K.A. McGarry, and M.G. Cyr. "Perioperative Care of the Patient with Hip Fracture." *Comprehensive Therapy* 29, no. 4 (Winter 2003): 233–43.

Tephly, T.R., and K.E. McMartin. "Methanol Metabolism and Toxicity in Aspartame." In *Physiology and Biochemistry*, edited by L.D. Stegink and L.J. Filer, Jr., 111. New York: Marcel Dekker, 1984.

Tucker, K.L., K. Morita, N. Qiao, M.T. Hannan, L.A. Cupples, and D.P. Kiel. "Colas, But Not Other Carbonated Beverages, Are Associated with Low Bone Mineral Density in Older Women: The Framingham Osteoporosis Study." *American Journal of Clinical Nutrition* 84, no. 4 (October 2006): 936–42.

Willett, Walter C. et al. "Health Professionals Follow-Up Study." Harvard School of Public Health, 2005. Available at: http://www.hsph.harvard.edu/hpfs.

Wykshak, G., and R.E. Frisch. "Carbonated Beverages, Dietary Calcium, the Dietary Calcium/Phosphorus Ratio, and Bone Fractures in Girls and Boys." *Journal of Adolescent Health* 15, no. 3 (May 1994): 210–15.

Young, Robert O., and Shelley Redford Young. *The pH Miracle for Diabetes: The Revolutionary Diet Plan for Type 1 and Type 2 Diabetics.* New York: Warner Books, 2004.

———. *The pH Miracle for Weight Loss: Balance Your Body Chemistry, Achieve Your Ideal Weight.* New York: Warner Books, 2006.

———. *Sick and Tired? Reclaim Your Inner Health.* Pleasant Grove, UT: Woodland Publishing, 2001.

Index

Note: Recipe titles are in **bold type**.